**Book Title:** Aid for Decontamination of Fire and Rescue Service Protective Clothing and Equipment After Chemical, Biological, and Radiological Exposures.

**Book Author:** James R. Lawson; T L. Jarboe

**Book Abstract:** The first priority for fire and rescue service personnel and all emergency first responders when responding to any call is the safety of all emergency personnel. Emergency first responders have been called to every recent terrorist attack in North America, and they will continue to be called since it is their job to assess the situation, establish control over the situation, and attempt to rescue people threatened by the attack. The threat of chemical, biological, radiological and nuclear (CBRN) attack is apparent, and all first responders must be prepared to address this possibility. This document provides the first responder with basic procedures for emergency decontamination of personal protective clothing and equipment (PPE) in the event that it is exposed to CBRN contamination. It also addresses processes for safely securing protective clothing and equipment that is considered to be unusable after a CBRN exposure. Some of the decontamination procedures addressed in this document are based on standard HAZMAT practices. In addition, information for normal care and cleaning of fire and rescue service PPE is included. This document has not been prepared to address decontamination processes for all known chemical or biological agents or radiological materials. It has been prepared to address approaches that may be used in emergency situations to decontaminate and/or secure PPE that has been exposed to the more common CBRN threats.

**Citation:** NIST SP - 981

**Keyword:** Biological; chemical; decontamination; fire fighter; first responder; hazmat; nuclear; personal protective clothing; radiological

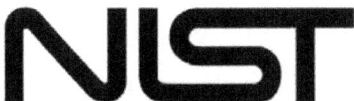

# National Institute of Standards and Technology

Technology Administration, U.S. Department of Commerce

*NIST Special Publication 981*

*Aid for Decontamination of Fire and Rescue Service Protective Clothing and Equipment After Chemical, Biological, and Radiological Exposures*

*J. Randall Lawson and Theodore L. Jarboe*

*NIST Special Publication 981*

# *Aid For Decontamination of Fire and Rescue Service Protective Clothing and Equipment After Chemical, Biological, and Radiological Exposures*

J. Randall Lawson

Building and Fire Research Laboratory
National Institute of Standards and Technology
Gaithersburg, MD 20899-0001

Theodore L. Jarboe

Bureau Chief / Fire Marshal
Montgomery County Fire and Rescue Service
Rockville, Maryland 20850

May 2002

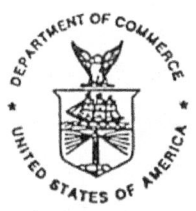
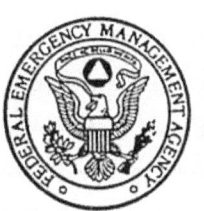
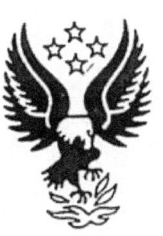

U.S. Department of Commerce
Donald L. Evans, *Secretary*
Technology Administration
Phillip J. Bond, *Under Secretary for Technology*
National Institute of Standards and Technology
Arden L. Bement, Jr., *Director*

Sponsored in part by:
Federal Emergency Management
Administration
Joe M. Allbaugh, *Director*
U.S. Fire Administration
R. David Paulison, *Administrator*

National Institute of Standards and Technology Special Publication 981
Natl. Inst. Stand. Technol. Spec. Publ. 981, 97 pages (May 2002)
CODEN: NSPUE2

U.S. GOVERNMENT PRINTING OFFICE
WASHINGTON: 2002

---

For sale by the Superintendent of Documents, U.S. Government Printing Office
Internet: bookstore.gpo.gov — Phone: (202) 512-1800 — Fax: (202) 512-2250
Mail: Stop SSOP, Washington, DC 20402-0001

# CONTENTS

## SCOPE

*This document has been prepared to provide all segments of the fire and rescue service and other emergency first responders with information for basic decontamination processes. It also provides methods for removing personal protective equipment (PPE) from service that may have been exposed to chemical or biological agents or radiological materials (CBRN) encountered during rescue attempts associated with a Weapons of Mass Destruction (WMD) attack. The document primarily addresses decontamination of PPE after low level exposures to CBRN agents or materials that would generally exist following an attack. Typically, a first responder would arrive on the scene some time after the primary attack, and the time between initiation of the attack and time of arrival will usually allow CBRN agents or materials to be diluted by air movement, weather conditions, or settle to the ground. Therefore, the first responder would not expect to be confronted with the maximum concentration of materials used during the attack. Where WMD attacks occur inside buildings, dangerous concentrations of agents or materials may exist in different parts of the building as a result of heating and air conditioning (HVAC) flows or other issues related to building ventilation. Also, some agents and materials are known to be persistent, and these agents or materials are sometimes recognizable by their residue. Persistent agents and materials may often be recognized as liquids, oily substances, dusts, and powders. In addition, first responders must be aware that terrorists may also target them in a second attack directed at eliminating rescue capability and attempt to degrade overall emergency response capabilities. In this case, first responders may become exposed to the maximum threat of an attack.*

*In the event of a high level exposure to CBRN agents or materials, this document will assist by providing some basic approaches for emergency decontamination if equipment must be available for immediate reuse. The document also provides methods for safely removing equipment from service that is considered to be unusable when applying available decontamination resources and when timely use of more advanced decontamination resources are not expected.*

*This document has not been prepared to address decontamination processes for all known chemical or biological agents or radiological materials. It has been prepared to address approaches that may be used in emergency situations to decontaminate and/or secure PPE that has been exposed to the more common CBRN threats.*

System of Units:

The policy of the National Institute of Standards and Technology is to use the International System of Units (metric or SI units) in all its publications as the primary set of units. However, in the American emergency services, non-SI units are so widely used instead of SI units that for clarity and usefulness, those customary and familiar units are used as the primary units in this document.

# Acknowledgements

The following people contributed to the development of this document:

Robert T. McCarthy and William J. Troup, United States Fire Administration, Federal Emergency Management Agency. The United States Fire Administration provided funding and technical assistance for the development of this document.

Dr. Richard Young, Senior Research Chemist, Dupont Advanced Fiber Systems

Charles L. Barber, Senior Technical Marketing Specialist, Dupont Advanced Fiber Systems

Robert L. Jensen, Jr., 3M , Minnesota Mining and Manufacturing Company, Safety and Security Systems Division

Peter L. Brown, Associate, W.L. Gore and Associates, Inc.

Daniel J. Gohlke, Product Specialist, W.L. Gore & Associates, Inc.

Don Aldridge, Vice-President, Fire Service Systems Research and Development, Lion Apparel

Karen Strumlock, Director of Resource Performance, Fire Service Systems Research and Development, Lion Apparel

Denise N. Statham, Director of Marketing, Southern Mills, Inc.

Sue Tribble, Sales Manager, Southern Mills, Inc.

Dr. Nadia S. El-Ayouby, Department of Health and Human Services, Centers for Disease Control and Prevention, NIOSH – ALOSH, National Personal Protective Laboratory

Robert D. McLaren, ITT Industries, Advanced Engineering and Sciences Division

Stephen M. Seltzer, NIST, Radiation Interactions and Dosimetry Group

Timothy F. Mengers, NIST Occupational Health and Safety Division, Health Physics

Judy L. Crain, NIST Occupational Health and Safety Division, Safety Office

Capt. J. W. Malinoski, MSC, U.S. Navy, Head, Radiation Sciences Department, Armed Forces Radiobiology Research Institute

Lt. Col. Horance Tsu, U.S. Air Force, MC, FS, Military Medical Operations, Armed Forces Radiobiology Research Institute

Lt. Matthew S. Welch, United States Marine Corps, Quantico, VA

Dr. Paul D. Fedele, Chief Scientist, MIRP, United States Army, Soldier and Biological Chemical Command, (SBCCOM)

Battalion Chief, Stephen J. King, III, Commander, Safety Battalion 1, Fire Department City of New York

Chief Thomas P. Rhodes, NIST, Facilities Services Division, Fire Protection Group (Fire Department)

Capt. Robert L. Vettori, Montgomery County Fire and Rescue Service, Montgomery County, MD

William H. Twilley, NIST, Fire Research Division, Fire Fighting Technology Group

Stephen Kerber, NIST, Fire Research Division, Fire Fighting Technology Group

Roy A. McLane, NIST, Fire Research Division, Materials Group

Dr. Barbara C. Levin, NIST, Biotechnology Division, Chemical Science and Technology Laboratory

Dr. Marcia J. Holden, NIST, Biotechnology Division, Chemical Science and Technology Laboratory

Aid for Decontamination of Fire And Rescue Service Protective Clothing and
Equipment After Chemical, Biological, and Radiological Exposures

by

J. Randall Lawson and Theodore L. Jarboe

Abstract

The first priority for fire and rescue service personnel and all emergency first responders
when responding to any call is the safety of all emergency personnel. Emergency first
responders have been called to every recent terrorist attack in North America, and they will
continue to be called since it is their job to assess the situation, establish control over the
situation, and attempt to rescue people threatened by the attack. The threat of chemical,
biological, radiological and nuclear (CBRN) attack is apparent, and all first responders must
be prepared to address this possibility. This document provides the first responder with basic
procedures for emergency decontamination of personal protective clothing and equipment
(PPE) in the event that it is exposed to CBRN contamination. It also addresses processes for
safely securing protective clothing and equipment that is considered to be unusable after a
CBRN exposure. Some of the decontamination procedures addressed in this document are
based on standard HAZMAT practices. In addition, information for normal care and
cleaning of fire and rescue service PPE is included. This document has not been prepared to
address decontamination processes for all known chemical or biological agents or
radiological materials. It has been prepared to address approaches that may be used in
emergency situations to decontaminate and/or secure PPE that has been exposed to the more
common CBRN threats.

Keywords: Biological, chemical, decontamination, fire fighter, first responder, hazmat,
nuclear, personal protective clothing, radiological

1

# Section I

# DECONTAMINATION BASICS

# 1.0  INTRODUCTION

Decontamination as defined for use in this document is: *the reduction or removal of chemical or biological agents, or radiological or nuclear materials (CBRN) so they are no longer hazards [1].*

*This document has not been prepared to provide methods for decontaminating protective clothing and equipment after exposures to all agent types or concentrations that exist.  It has been prepared to give some basic guidelines for handling equipment that has been exposed to relatively low concentration CBRN environments where human rescue is practical when using NFPA 1971 [2] compliant structural fire fighting ensembles.  The document is designed to provide the first responder with useful information to assist in making decisions related to emergency decontamination and removing equipment from service that has been exposed to low concentration CBRN environments.*

*Circumstances at the scene of a weapon of mass destruction (WMD) incident may dictate that the Incident Commander must alter procedures recommended in this aid so that specific needs may be addressed.*

The most important safety issue for fire and rescue service personnel responding to a call for assistance is the safety of all personnel responding to the call.  Failure to take this important factor into account can result in first responder injuries or loss of life.  In these cases, the response of fire and rescue service personnel to the call becomes an effort to save members of their own units and distracts from the primary goal of assisting others that need help.  The safety of fire and rescue service personnel is an important factor in every dispatch, whether it is for a house fire, automobile accident, or terrorist attack.  A problem with a terrorist attack as compared to a typical incident is that terrorist attacks may be much more poorly defined, and the attack may also be targeting the first responders as they arrive on the scene.  When chemical, biological or radiological agents or materials are used in a weapon of mass destruction attack, the potential for personnel and equipment exposure to hazardous environments may be great.  Exposures of first responders and their equipment to hostile CBRN environments may have a significant short term and long term impact on their ability to assist victims that need help.  However in many of these situations, it is likely that the first responders will arrive after the release of life threatening toxic agents or materials.  As a result of time and varying environmental conditions, it also is likely that the concentration of the agent (except for persistent agents) may be greatly diminished upon arriving at the scene.  However, even small exposures of personnel and equipment to life threatening CBRN environments bring with them serious questions concerning the ability of the responders and their equipment to safely function on calls that follow the initial event.  If personnel and their equipment become contaminated the question becomes, what must be done to protect the personnel, and how can the equipment be decontaminated so that it may be used during another incident that immediately follows.

*Currently, most fire departments don't have the resources that allow for excess equipment that can be discarded in the event that it becomes contaminated by CBRN agents or materials.  The loss of personnel and critical equipment to CBRN events quickly prevents the first responders from accomplishing their primary role, assisting others that are in danger. This situation becomes much more significant if terrorist attacks have been designed specifically to compromise the CBRN response capabilities of large fire departments and metropolitan rescue services or the attacks take advantage of the diminished CBRN response capabilities that are likely to exist in smaller communities. In many situations, CBRN support may take long periods of time to arrive when action by the local first responders could save lives and stabilize the threat. When any CBRN response capability has been compromised or eliminated and immediate backup is not available, the average first responder must be prepared to provide assistance to victims and be able to assist in stabilizing events at the incident.*

This document has been prepared to provide a single reference source for assisting the emergency first responder with decision making for decontamination and securing of protective clothing and equipment items after CBRN exposures. Currently, there is no single source of information that provides a broad base of information on decontamination of fire service protective ensembles that have been exposed to CBRN agents. Some information is available through the National Fire Protection Association (NFPA) standards for hazardous materials (HAZMAT) operations. Additional information is provided by the United States Centers for Disease Control and Prevention (CDC); National Institute for Occupational Safety and Health (NIOSH); the United States Environmental Protection Agency (EPA); the United States Army Soldier and Biological Chemical Command (SBCCOM); and various equipment manufacturers.

## 2.0 NORMAL CARE AND CLEANING

Recommended care and cleaning procedures for fire fighters' protective clothing ensembles is contained in NFPA 1851, Standard on Selection, Care, and Maintenance of Structural Fire Fighting Protective Ensembles [3]. The first edition of this standard was published in 2001. This NFPA standard includes information on cleaning of protective garments (coats and pants), helmets, gloves, footwear, and hoods. Cleaning and decontamination procedures for typical fire service equipment exposures are contained in Chapter 5 of the standard. *The___ NFPA 1851 standard does not include cleaning and decontamination procedures for CBRN exposures.* However, it is recommended that a copy of the standard be obtained from NFPA and bound with this document. Chapter 5 of NFPA 1851 includes sections on routine cleaning, advanced cleaning, specialized cleaning, and cleaning and decontamination procedures. Procedures described include utility sink and machine cleaning. *When using the NFPA 1851 document, it is important to understand the definitions: "biological agent" and "hazardous materials".* It must be remembered that these definitions as applied in the standard primarily relate to operations where typical fire service exposures occur and do not relate to WMD events [4]. When the NFPA document was written, the biological agent definition was prepared as it related to potential exposure to human body fluids from individuals with life threatening diseases. This definition did not include the concept of intentional releases of chemical or biological warfare agents, toxic industrial chemicals, or radiological materials. Also, the types of HAZMAT exposures addressed by the standard primarily relate to incidental exposures to common industrial or agricultural chemicals and are typically not associated with major hazardous materials exposures where specialized HAZMAT equipment is required.

## 3.0 CHEMICAL, BIOLOGICAL, AND RADIOLOGICAL ENVIRONMENTS

It is common that terrorist attacks are often made using single methods of attack like explosives, chemical, or biological agents. This is demonstrated by the attacks on the World Trade Center, the Sarin (GB) attack in Japan, and the release of anthrax in the United States mail. This is not the only way that an attack may occur. In a weapons of mass destruction attack multiple threats should be expected. Review of terrorist attack scenarios show that they often refer to the use of multiple threats that include explosives (conventional and nuclear), incendiaries, chemical agents, biological agents, and radiological materials. As a result, emergency first responders must be knowledgeable about these threats. Of these threats, the more subtle forms may appear to be nothing more than a condition that resembles the release of carbon monoxide by poorly maintained heating equipment or it could take on the form of conditions that occur during a common structural fire. A clue to recognizing these subtle forms of attack is that they threaten numerous people, critical components of public or defense infrastructure, and/or symbolic targets: e.g., Statue of Liberty, or Washington Monument.

This section and following sections characterize some of the more common chemical, biological, and radiological threats. Each section contains basic information on the threat and where possible provides the information in the form of easily used tables[1].

## 3.1 COMMON PRACTICES FOR EMERGENCY CBRN DECONTAMINATION

There are some practices that are common for immediate emergency decontamination of first responder's PPE upon exposure to CBRN agents and materials. Although exposures to biological agents or radiological materials may not require immediate gross decontamination of personnel, it may require that PPE be decontaminated and maintained in a state ready for use after an initial event. The following is a list of common practices used for establishing emergency field decontamination stations for first responders PPE [5]:

Important Note: *Where possible, emergency decontamination areas and corridors for first responders should be set up separate from mass decontamination areas for the public. This is because first responder decontamination processes are a working part of the emergency response and may require different procedures and management considerations from those represented by mass decontamination for the public.*

The primary objective of decontamination is to avoid contaminating anyone or anything beyond the hot zone. When in doubt always decontaminate personnel, equipment and apparatus [6] unless it is to remain in the hot zone for reuse.

---

[1] *This document contains text that provides warnings and critical information related to given topics. These warnings and critical information are written in bold, or italics, and are signified by the following words written in bold type*: Warning or Important Note

### 3.1.1 DECONTAMINATION AREA AND CORRIDOR

The following describes how to prepare decontamination areas and corridors at suspected WMD attack sites: See decontamination area location diagrams. (Figure 1 and 2)

1. Position decontamination area upwind and uphill of suspected hazard areas. If possible, position the decontamination areas so water runoff can be collected for removal and treatment. If this is not possible water runoff should be directed so it will collect in a grassy or soil area. Locate decontamination areas so that water from decontamination does not flow into casualty or work areas. *In an emergency decontamination setting, life safety takes precedence over containing runoff [5].*

2. Mark off a decontamination area with two parts. The two parts should be located adjacent and parallel to each other. One side is the decontamination corridor, and the other side is the decontamination area.

3. The decontamination area is divided into two parts. One part should be uphill and upwind of the lower part.

4. A personnel entry area located on the hot zone side at the base of the decontamination corridor, and it should be positioned so that personnel do not stand in contaminated liquids flowing away from the decontamination area.

5. Make up a solution of detergent and water and obtain soft scrub brushes. Scrub brushes are not to be used on the skin.

6. Prepare a reserve air supply, preferably with a workline unit or spare Self-Contained Breathing Apparatus (SCBA)s and/or cylinders.

7. If possible, place an impermeable (e.g., polyethylene) sheet, weighted down at the edges, at the exit point of the uphill decontamination area.

8. The decontamination crew will don SCBA and, where available, disposable chemical suits.

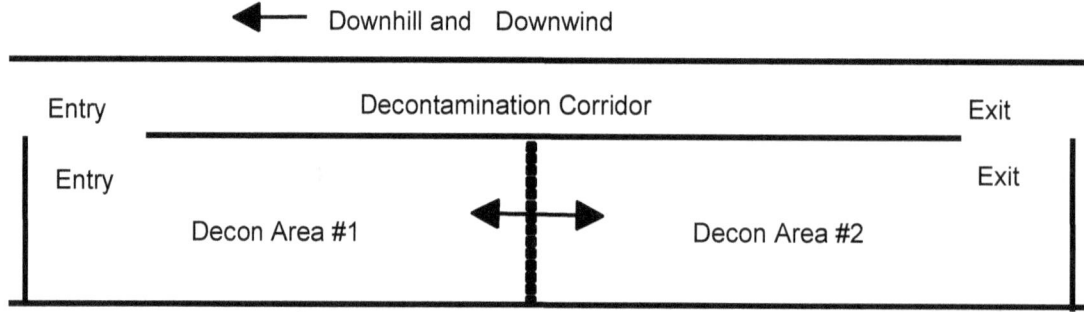

Figure 1. Decontamination area layout

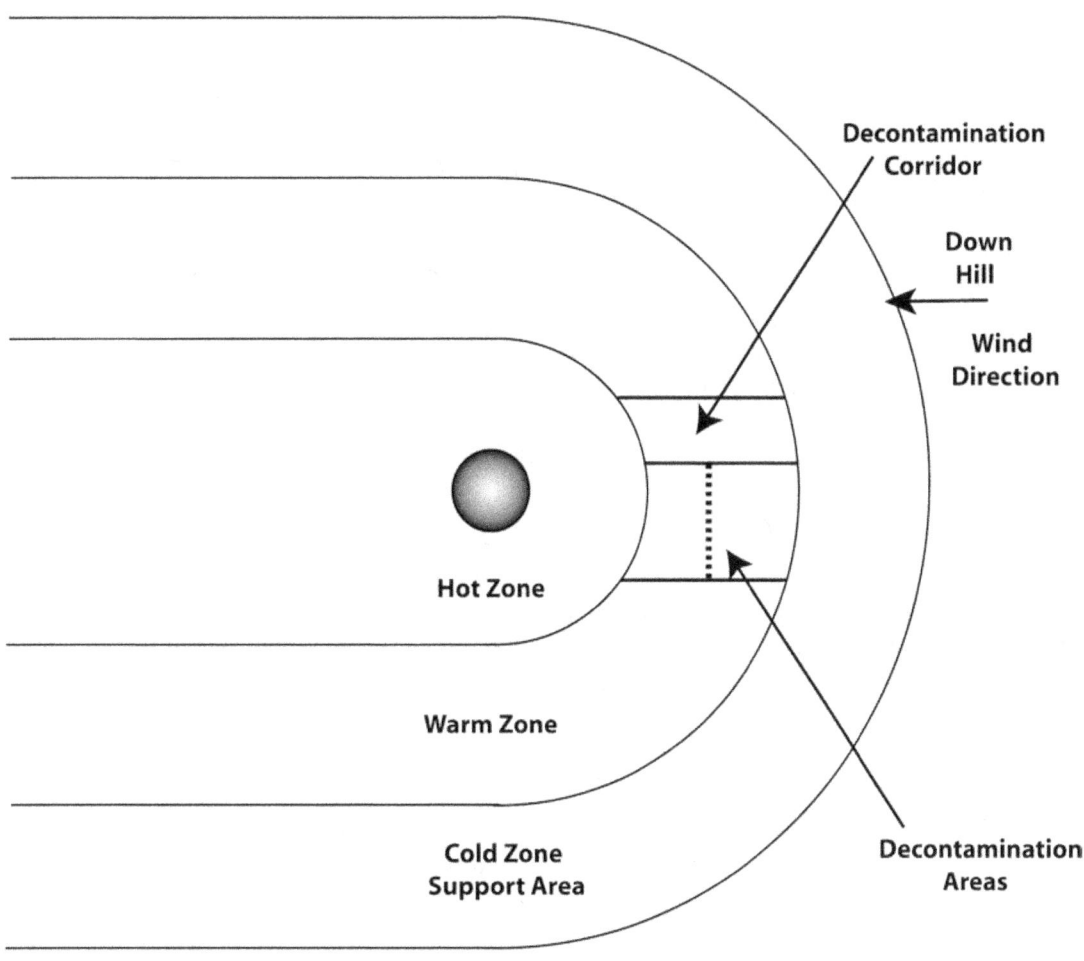

Figure 2.  Decontamination area location

## 3.1.2 DECONTAMINATION IN COLD ENVIRONMENTS

Cold environments create problems related to decontamination.  The most important is that personnel being decontaminated are subject to hypothermia and cold shock.  In very cold environments water used for decontamination will freeze and seriously limit decontamination processes.  In weather conditions where the air temperature is 65 °F (18 °C) or colder, efforts must be made to keep personnel warm.  When temperatures are 35 °F (2 °C) or lower decontamination must be done in a heated building or shelter.  In conditions where structures are used as decontamination areas, decontamination triage should be done outside of the building.  In addition, wiping and blotting decontamination can be accomplished outside in low temperature environments, and personnel can remove clothing and bag it as they move into the building for body decontamination.

## 3.2 CHEMICAL METHODS FOR DECONTAMINATION

As mentioned above, large quantities of low pressure water is a primary cleaning solution that may be used for decontamination. Water not only dilutes and flushes CBRN agents and materials away, it will also react with many chemical warfare agents chemically to detoxify them. There are two other chemical decontamination processes easily used by first responders to neutralize chemical warfare (CWA) and biological warfare agents (BWA) and have also been recommended for radioactive materials decontamination [1][7]. These processes take advantage of common household materials that can easily be obtained from grocery stores, hardware stores, and swimming pool supply stores. These two methods are: 1) washing contaminated equipment with high pH, alkaline, soap solutions and 2) washing or soaking contaminated equipment with bleach solutions; calcium hypochlorite, $Ca(OCl)_2 + 2H_2O$, or sodium hypochlorite, $NaOCl + H_2O$ [1].

## 3.2.1 IMPORTANCE OF pH IN DECONTAMINATION

pH is a measure of the acidity or alkalinity of a solution. Chemically, acids and alkaline (base) solutions are opposites. The pH scale extends from 1, representing the strongest acids, to 14 representing the strongest alkaline or base solutions [8]. A neutral solution has a pH of 7. It is interesting to note that the intervals on the pH scale are exponential, and therefore represent vastly greater differences in solution concentrations than the numerical figures of the scale indicate. Many soaps are made with alkaline materials, including sodium hydroxide, NaOH, and potassium hydroxide, KOH. Sodium hydroxide (lye) is a common material found in grocery stores, home centers, and hardware stores (e.g. Drano etc.). It is often used as a drain and metal cleaner. Also, sea water is typically alkaline with pH values that range from 8 to 10.

Important Note:     *All fire fighting apparatus should have on board equipment that can be quickly and easily used for measuring pH of chemical decontamination solutions, and personnel should be trained to use the equipment for preparing decontamination solutions. Very inexpensive pH test kits contain paper test strips (litmus paper) that change color when exposed to various levels of acid or alkaline solutions. Paper test strips have a limited shelf life. In addition, relatively new and inexpensive handheld electronic pH meters are also available. These electronic instruments generally provide greater measurement resolution.*

Soap or detergent solutions that are prepared for decontamination of CW and BW agents should have a pH value of at least 8. If the soap solution shows a neutral (7 pH), the solution pH can be boosted by slowly adding lye and mixing it into the solution. The rate of detoxification increases sharply with pH values higher than 8 and increases by a factor of four for every 18 °F (10 °C) rise in temperature for the decontamination solution [9] [10]. The solution concentration should not exceed a pH value of 10.5.

Warning: *One must use caution when working with concentrated alkaline materials like lye. These materials in concentrated forms can cause serious injuries to the eyes and skin. They are hazardous materials. Follow manufacturer's directions and warnings listed on the container labels.*

## 3.2.2 PREPARING CHLORINE BLEACH SOLUTIONS

Chlorine bleach solutions are commonly used for detoxifying chemical warfare agents and decontaminating biological warfare agents. The following procedures give guidance on preparing the chlorine bleach solution that are most commonly used.

*Exercise caution when handling and storing chlorine bleach solutions. Household chlorine bleach is a corrosive substance and will react with metal containers and may produce an exothermic or heat generating reaction that may lead to ignition when in contact with fuels or solvents [6]. Common household bleach solutions as purchased from the grocery store may also injure human skin. Observe manufacturer's warnings and safety instructions listed on the product container.* Chlorine bleach products are affected by exposure to sunlight. However, when shielded from sunlight and stored in a closed container the product will only degrade about 1 % per year, i.e. from 6 % to 5 % [6]. Chlorine bleach solutions degrade faster in elevated temperatures and slower in colder temperature environments. Bleach containers become hard and easily crack with age. It is recommended that prepared bleach solutions be stored in new, unused, thick plastic, gasoline containers that have been well marked to identify the contents and safety information [6].

## CALCIUM HYPOCHLORITE BLEACH

One of the most common forms of calcium hypochlorite bleach is used as a swimming pool and spa sanitizer. Granular calcium hypochlorite containing 68 % available chlorine (HTH, manufactured by the Olin Corporation, Norwalk, CT or equivalent products) may be located at swimming pool supply stores and some hardware stores.
Warning: *Calcium hypochlorite (HTH) in its concentrated form is highly reactive and will burn on contact with the VX nerve agent [11].* It will also give off toxic vapors on contact with G agents and will burn the skin and destroy clothing [11]. Therefore, it should be used carefully. However, when properly mixed and properly applied, it is a highly effective material for decontaminating personnel, equipment, and surface-areas [11].

The following are suggested formulations that may be used for decontaminating CWA and BWA releases [11]: Swimming pool or spa sanitizer materials may be manufactured with varying amounts of calcium hypochlorite, and they may be manufactured to dissolve at different rates. Only the granular forms of calcium hypochlorite containing 68% available chlorine are addressed in this document. Pool sanitizer products are also manufactured into tablets and capsules.

Solutions for decontaminating of Chemical Warfare Agents (CWA) and Biological Warfare Agents (BWA), made with 68 % available chlorine calcium hypochlorite bleach:

Equipment decontamination [11]: 5 % solution for CWA. Add 5 lb (2268 g) of HTH to 12 gal (45.6 L) of water and carefully mix until completely blended.

11

Personnel decontamination [11]:  0.5 % solution for CWA and BWA.  Add 0.5 lb (227 g) of HTH to 12 gal (45.6 L) of water and carefully mix until completely blended.

Equipment decontamination [11]:  2 % solution for BWA.  Add 1 lb (454 g) of HTH to 6 gal (22.8 L) of water and carefully mix until completely blended.

SODIUM HYPOCHLORITE BLEACH

Note:  *Ultra chlorine bleach products found in grocery stores, with a 6 % sodium hypochlorite concentration typically has a pH of about 11.*

Preparing a 0.26 % chlorine bleach decontamination solution using 6.0 % sodium hypochlorite household bleach, Ultra Clorox® regular bleach or an equivalent product. Finished product is a (1:23) solution:

- *Obtain a container for mixing the decontamination solution, that does not leak, and easily holds at least 25 liquid measures (examples, 25 gal or 25 L)*

  Note:  *To expedite the mixing process, the water level and chlorine bleach levels may be pre-marked on the inside of the mixing container.  This is done by placing 22 liquid measures of clean water into the mixing container, and then clearly mark the water liquid level on the inside of the container.  Add 1 additional liquid measure to the mixing container, and mark the liquid level again.  This identifies the total liquid level after the ultra chlorine bleach has been added to the mixing container.*

- *Pour  22 measures (examples, gallons or liters) of clean water into the mixing container.  If the mixing container was pre-marked, fill to the "22 parts" level mark. Always fill container first with water, and then add the bleach solution.*

- *Pour 1 measure of 6.0 % ultra chlorine bleach into the mixing container.  If the mixing container was pre-marked, pour the bleach into the container until the liquid level reaches the top mark.*

Preparing a 0.5 % chlorine bleach decontamination solution using 6.0 % sodium hypochlorite household bleach, Ultra Clorox® regular bleach or an equivalent product.  Finished product is a (1:12) solution:

- *Obtain a container for mixing the decontamination solution, that does not leak, and easily holds at least 15 liquid measures (examples, 15 gal or 15 L)*

  Note:  *To expedite the mixing process, the water level and chlorine bleach levels may be pre-marked on the inside of the mixing container.  This is done by placing 11 liquid measures of clean water into the mixing container, and then clearly mark the water liquid level on the inside of the container.  Add 1 additional liquid measure to the mixing container, and mark the liquid level again.  This identifies the total liquid level after the bleach has been added to the mixing container.*

- *Pour 11 measures (examples, gallons or liters) of clean water into the mixing container. If the mixing container was pre-marked, fill to the "11 parts" level mark.*

- *Pour 1 measure of 6.0 % ultra chlorine bleach into the mixing container. If the mixing container was pre-marked, pour the bleach into the container until it reaches the top mark.*

Another commonly used decontamination solution is made from a 5.0 % sodium hypochlorite household bleach. This solution is often used in medical facilities as a disinfectant where dangerous infectious diseases are present [12].

Preparing a 0.5 % (1:10) chlorine bleach decontamination solution using a 5.0 % sodium hypochlorite household bleach:

- *Obtain a container for mixing the decontamination solution, that does not leak, and will easily hold 15 liquid measures (examples, 15 gal or 15 L)*

  Note: *As above, to expedite the mixing process the water level and chlorine bleach levels may be pre-marked on the inside of the mixing container. This is done by placing 9 liquid measures of clean water into the mixing container, and then clearly mark the "9 parts" liquid level on the inside of the container. Add 1 addition liquid measure to the mixing container, and mark the liquid level again. This identifies the total liquid level "10 parts" after the household chlorine bleach has been added to the container.*

Some household bleach products contain only 5.0 % sodium hypochlorite. These products may also contain other ingredients beneficial for home laundry processes, and little is known about how fire fighters' protective clothing and equipment will be affected by these other ingredients. The following describes how to prepare a 0.5 % (1:10) sodium hypochlorite decontamination solution when using household bleach products that contain 5.0 % sodium hypochlorite.

Making the 0.5% (1:10) solution:

- *Pour 9 measures (examples, gallons or liters) of clean water into the mixing container. If the mixing container was pre-marked, fill to the "9 parts" level mark.*

- *Pour 1 measure of 5.0 % sodium hypochlorite household bleach into the mixing container. If the mixing container was pre-marked, pour the commercial bleach into the container until it reaches the top mark.*

### 3.2.3 COMMON DECONTAMINATION METHODS

### DECONTAMINATION USING POOL AND SPA SANITIZERS

The following 68 % available chlorine calcium hypochlorite solutions (HTH or equivalent) are suggested for decontaminating CWA and BWA agents [11]:

Warning: *No information is available on the potential harmful effects that pool and spa sanitizing solutions may have on first responders' personal protective clothing and equipment. To determine the potential for damage, pretest solutions on old gear that is being decommissioned.*

Personnel decontamination [11]: 0.5 % calcium hypochlorite solution as prepared in Section 3.2.2, for CWA and BWA, 15 minute contact time followed by a thorough rinse with clean tepid water.

Equipment decontamination [11]: 5 % calcium hypochlorite solution as prepared in Section 3.2.2, for CWA, 15 minute contact time followed by a thorough rinse with clean tepid water.

Equipment decontamination [11]: 2 % calcium hypochlorite solution as prepared in Section 3.2.2, for BWA, 15 minute contact time followed by a thorough rinse with clean tepid water.

EMERGENCY DECONTAMINATION USING 6 % CHLORINE BLEACH

Warning : *This treatment is for emergency decontamination only and should be used only one time on materials containing Kevlar®. See Section 4, page 16.*

- Completely soak the protective clothing and equipment for one minute in undiluted Ultra Clorox® regular bleach or an equivalent product that contains a 6 % sodium hypochlorite solution.
- Do not dilute the manufacturer's bleach solution with water, as is normally done.
- After the one minute soak in the ultra chlorine bleach solution, immediately rinse the protective clothing with large quantities of tepid water. Air dry or use appropriate machine drying processes.

*Note: Some materials may show a change in color.*

Warning : *For Kevlar® containing fabrics, repeated exposures to chlorine containing solutions will result in serious loss of material strength and will cause the protective clothing systems to fail when in normal use. See Section 4, page 16.*

NORMAL DECONTAMINATION USING 6 % CHLORINE BLEACH

Use on fire fighters' protective clothing and equipment that does not contain materials that are seriously degraded by exposure to chlorine solutions.

This process may be used on protective equipment that does not contain Kevlar® and has firm or hard equipment surfaces: Examples: helmets, rubber boots, some gloves, SCBA tanks and harness frames, masks, rubber hoses, and external regulator surfaces.

Warning : *Check with your SCBA manufacturer for decontamination procedures for internal components of SCBA regulators and masks.*

- Completely soak the protective clothing and equipment for 15 minute in a household bleach (sodium hypochlorite) solution that has been diluted to produce a 0.26 % (1:22) bleach solution.
- After the 15 minute soak in the 1:22 bleach solution, immediately rinse the protective clothing and equipment with large quantities of tepid water.

## PHYSICAL METHODS FOR CHEMICAL AND BIOLOGICAL WARFARE AGENT DECONTAMINATION.

Fire fighters' protective ensembles that meet the requirements of the NFPA 1971 standard [2] must pass a test for "Heat and Thermal Shrinkage Resistance." This test exposes ensemble components to an oven test to determine if the materials will degrade when exposed for five minutes to an oven temperature of 260 °C (500 °F). The test requires that the materials must not ignite, melt, drip, or separate following the exposure. In addition, the materials must not exhibit excessive shrinkage after the exposure. Requirements for this standard, as well as research results from other studies, indicate that the fire fighters' protective ensemble should withstand the dry heat exposures listed below for chemical and biological agent decontamination. Steam heat (autoclaving) may also be used to decontaminate biological contamination. The steam method is discussed in Section I, 4.2 and in Section IV.

## DRY HEAT METHOD:

Heat combined with clean air circulation and venting will evaporate most chemical agents after decontamination blotting, flushing, and washing has been completed. After the materials have been dried at the elevated temperatures recommended below, they may be washed using the procedures specified in NFPA 1851 [3].

Expose biologically contaminated materials to one of the following temperature/time conditions [1]:

> *180 °C (356 °F) for ................30 minutes*
> *170 °C (340 °F) for .............1 hour*
> *160 °C (320 °F) for............... 2 hours.*
> *150 °C (300 °F) for ..............2.5 hours*

Some fire training facilities have live fire training compartments that may be adapted for the above dry heat method of decontamination. It is critical that all components and parts of the materials being decontaminated reach the recommended dry heat temperature, and they must be maintained at the given temperature for at least the specified time period.

## 3.3 SECURING AND DISPOSAL OF EQUIPMENT

In cases where protective clothing and equipment have been contaminated with high concentrations of chemical or biological agents, or radiological materials, and damaged during operations, it is likely that the items will have to be secured to prevent the spread of the contamination. In addition when protective clothing and equipment can not be decontaminated, it will also need to be secured. Methods for securing contaminated materials are addressed in each of the following sections for the different CBRN threats.

Items useful for securing contaminated equipment [6]:

- Heavy gauge, 6 mil (0.15 mm) thick or thicker, plastic garbage bags, large enough to be used as a drum-liner bag. Clear bags are more useful than opaque colored bags since they permit identification of contents without opening the bag.

- Identification tags to mark each bag and drum of contaminated equipment.

- Indelible marking pens for preparing identification tags.

- Clean steel drums with full drum diameter lids that can be removed for inserting bags of contaminated equipment. Lids must be capable of being removed and placed back on the drum and sealed.

## 4.0 IMPACT OF DECONTAMINATION ON PPE

Little information is available concerning the impact that decontamination processes have on the performance of personal protective clothing and equipment. Limited preliminary work by industry and NIST is beginning to provide some understanding. Several product manufacturers have supplied preliminary test data on the performance of their products after being exposed to decontamination methods using sodium hypochlorite-based bleach solutions, and NIST has replicated some of this work. These initial data provide a mix of results. The following briefly describes these preliminary findings:

The preliminary studies involved the following materials that are commonly used to fabricate protective clothing for first responders:

| Material* | Use |
|---|---|
| Aralite® | Thermal Liner |
| Three Layer Nomex®E-89 | Thermal Liner |
| Nomex® III-Defender™ | Outer Shell Fabric |
| Nomex® IIIA | Outer Shell and Moisture Barrier Substrate |
| PBI™ -Kevlar® Kombat™ | Outer Shell Fabric |
| Nomex® Kevlar®Advanced™ | Outer Shell Fabric |
| Kevlar®/ Nomex® | Outer Shell Fabric |
| Nomex® E-89 Crosstech® | Moisture Barrier  E-89, Discontinued by Gore 2001 |
| Nomex® IIIA Pajama Check-Crosstech® | Moisture Barrier |
| Scotchlite® Fire Coat Trim Materials | Reflective Trim |

* Advanced™, Aralite®, Defender™, and Kombat™ are registered trademarks of Southern Mills.
   Nomex®, and Kevlar® are registered trademarks of E.I. Dupont.
   PBI™ is a registered trademark of Celanese Corporation
   Crosstech® is a registered trademark of W.L. Gore & Associates
   Scotchlite® is a registered trademark of 3M, Minnesota Mining and Manufacturing Company

The preliminary studies investigated whether the above products experience tensile strength changes after being exposed to two recommended procedures for decontamination that use commercial sodium hypochlorite bleach solutions. These preliminary studies are limited in scope; however performance trends for the above products are evident.

## 4.1 IMPACT OF CHEMICAL DECONTAMINATION METHODS ON PPE

The experimental procedure included the following: All the materials were new. They were all pre-washed one time using a home machine laundry (Machine cycle 1, AATCC 135) method [13]. No ballast was used. The materials were dried using a typical home electric clothes dryer using a standard drying cycle. After the materials were dry, half of the specimens were immediately tested in a laboratory tensile strength test machine while following ASTM D5034 for breaking strength [13]. The other half of the specimens was treated to one of the two recommended decontamination procedures:

Procedure 1: Soak individual specimens in a 6 % sodium hypochlorite bleach solution for one minute, and immediately rinse the specimens in tap water.

Procedure 2: Soak individual specimens in a 1:20 sodium hypochlorite bleach solution for 15 minutes, and immediately rinse the specimens in tap water.

In general, from this limited set of data, all except one of the materials listed above showed no loss of tensile strength or only a slight loss of tensile strength after a single exposure to Procedure 1. The only material that showed a significant difference in breaking strength was the Nomex® E-89 Crosstech® moisture barrier. (W.L. Gore stopped producing this material in 2001.) This material showed only a slight change in physical appearance; however, it did tend to stretch more than the untreated material. One of the manufacturer's studies had results from "Procedure 1" and also results from studies that extended bleach soak times by one minute increments until they reached a maximum soak time of five minutes. These preliminary results showed that materials containing Kevlar ® had a noticeable loss in tensile strength as soak time in the bleach increased. However, none of the materials showed catastrophic tensile strength loss even with the five minute soak time. Information from this manufacturer's study did not include the Nomex ® E-89 Crosstech® moisture barrier. None of the materials exhibited any discoloration noticeable to the eye following exposure to either Procedure 1 or Procedure 2.

Greater differences were noted with some materials after being exposed to decontamination Procedure 2. A trend is apparent that materials containing Kevlar ® are affected by longer exposures to a 1:20 bleach solution, and strength continues to be lost with each repeated exposure to Procedure 2 until the Kevlar ® is dissolved and removed from the material. Of the shell materials, only the materials primarily composed of Nomex ® showed little or no change in strength after repeated exposures to Procedure 2. Another set of products that showed little or no change in strength, reflective quality, or surface appearance was the range of Scotchlite® Fire Coat Trim materials.

Other disinfecting products have been tested to determine if they will degrade aramid materials such as Nomex ® and Kevlar ®. However, the aramid fiber manufacturer did not have data regarding the value of the products as a disinfectant. These disinfecting products that did not damage aramid fabrics are listed in the Appendix A. In addition, the Appendix A contains preliminary information on the Modec Decon Formulation, developed by Sandia National Laboratories.

## 4.2 IMPACT OF THERMAL DECONTAMINATION METHODS ON PPE

There are two thermal methods for decontaminating personal protective clothing and equipment discussed in Section IV, 1.0, page 45. One is a dry heat method and the second is a steam heat method, autoclaving. Again, preliminary tests have been conducted to determine if a materials tensile strength would degrade if exposed to the decontamination procedures.

## DRY HEAT DECONTAMINATION

The following dry heat experimental procedure was used: The same materials addressed above in the chemical study were used in this study. The most challenging thermal exposure condition was used in this preliminary study. The materials were pre-washed and dried using the procedure mentioned above [13]. This limited study exposed three specimens of each material to the 180 °C (356 °F) oven environments for a period of 30 minutes. The materials were allowed to cool, and then they were tested for tensile strength using the ASTM D5034 procedure [14].

Results from this limited study showed that only one of the materials experienced a decrease in tensile strength after the thermal exposure. This tensile strength loss was again experienced with the Nomex ® E89 Crosstech ® moisture barrier. These preliminary data suggest that the other materials showed no significant changes in tensile strength, and no visual changes in physical characteristics were observed in the successful materials after the thermal exposure.

## STEAM HEAT DECONTAMINATION (AUTOCLAVE)

The following steam heat experimental procedure was used: The same materials addressed above in the chemical study and dry heat study were used. The materials were pre-washed and dried using the procedure mentioned above [13]. This limited study exposed at three specimens of each material to the following minimum autoclave conditions: 121 °C ± 2 °C (250 °F ± 4 °F), minimum one atmosphere pressure above ambient, for a time period of 20 minutes. The materials were allowed to cool, and then they were tested for tensile strength using the ASTM D5034 procedure [14].

Results from this preliminary study exhibited the same trends in tensile strength shown by the dry heat decontamination method. Tensile strength loss was again experienced with the Nomex® E89 Crosstech ® moisture barrier. Again, with this limited data set, the other materials showed no significant changes in tensile strength, and no visual changes in physical characteristics were observed after the thermal exposure.

USEFUL REFERENCE SOURCES

Guide for the Selection of Chemical and Biological Decontamination Equipment for Emergency First Responders, NIJ Guide 103-00, National Institute of Justice, Office of Law Enforcement Standards, National Institute of Standards and Technology, Department of Defense Technical Information Center.

Guide for the Selection of Chemical Agent and Toxic Industrial Material Detection Equipment for Emergency First Responders, NIJ Guide 100-00, , National Institute of Justice, Office of Law Enforcement Standards, National Institute of Standards and Technology, Department of Defense Technical Information Center, June 2000.

# Section II

# EMERGENCY DECONTAMINATION OF INJURED PERSONNEL

## II. EMERGENCY DECONTAMINATION OF INJURED PERSONNEL

In the event that a first responder becomes contaminated and is experiencing toxic effects from a chemical agent and/or becomes seriously injured at the scene, they should be decontaminated before being transported for further medical care. The procedures listed below give guidance on emergency decontamination of injured personnel. These procedures are based on recommendations provided in the NFPA, Hazardous Materials Response Handbook [6]:

Important Note: *In cases where radioactive materials are present and the level of environmental radiological exposure is manageable, it is emphasized that the contamination on the victim presents little or no danger to the responder rendering necessary first-aid, even if the victim has not been fully and properly decontaminated. Proper first-aid should ALWAYS be administered [15]. However, efforts should be made to decontaminate victims before being transported for further medical care.*

For radioactive materials incidents: *It is important that life-saving procedures take precedence over decontamination. "Treatment of life-threatening injuries, e.g., severe trauma, shock, hemorrhage, and respiratory distress, always takes precedence over decontamination procedures, treatment of possible symptoms from irradiation, and dose estimation procedures." [7]*

1. For cases where radioactive materials may be present, carefully scan personnel with a radiation monitor suitable for detecting surface contamination. All parts of their protective clothing and equipment will be scanned, including the soles of boots. If no reading above normal background level is measured and no other contamination is observed or suspected, the person can leave the decontamination area through a safe corridor.

2. For contaminated personnel. Remove the person from the contaminated area and into a decontamination area. Be sure that the person has adequate breathing air. If the air supply is low, provide the individual with an adequate supply of uncontaminated breathing air or oxygen.

3. Be careful not to break the victim's skin during the decontamination process. In the event that the victim has open wounds, cover them, and be careful that the decontamination process does not cause additional contamination of the wounds.

4. If nuclear or radioactive materials are involved, monitor the person for radiological contamination and remove those parts of clothing that are contaminated.

5. Remove the helmet and immediately wash all chemical or biological contaminated areas and/or radiological hot spots down with copious amounts of low pressure water. Blot concentrations of chemical agents that are not being removed by flushing and continue flushing. Flush all exposed parts of the body that may have been contaminated.

6.  If the victim is wearing SCBA, leave the mask in place and sealed, release the harness, and remove the tank and harness. Remove and replace breathing air connections and hoses as needed, but be sure that the victim has a safe, clean, and adequate breathing air supply as the decontamination process is taking place.

7.  Remove all contaminated clothing, if necessary by cutting it off the victim. Be careful to prevent the victim from having further contact with any contamination. Continue washing any skin contamination of the victim while clothing removal is in progress. A 0.5 % hypochlorite bleach solution may be used for washing followed by a clean tepid water rinse.

8.  Cover the victim to prevent shock and loss of body heat.

9.  Move the victim to a safe clean area. Provide emergency medical care as required, but do not apply mouth-to-mouth resuscitation. Bag masks and mechanical ventilation may be used. Be careful that contamination does not enter the mouth or airways.

10. Send victim for immediate medical treatment as soon as emergency decontamination is completed. In radiological cases, complete decontamination may not be necessary before transporting the victim. However, it is important that the victim is wrapped or placed into a protective cover such as a large plastic bag to prevent spread of contamination.

11. Ensure that the ambulance personnel and hospital are informed that the victim has been contaminated and that the victim only received emergency decontamination.

# Section III

# CHEMICAL WARFARE INCIDENTS

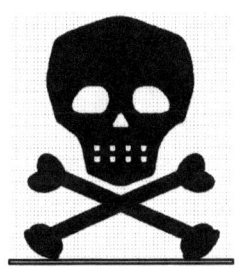

*Chemical Agent Symbol*

## III. CHEMICAL WARFARE AGENTS AND TOXIC INDUSTRIAL CHEMICALS

Chemical threats may be broken down into four general categories: nerve agents (G and V), blister agents (H and L), blood agents and choking agents. These agents can be dispersed in the air we breathe, in the water we drink, or on surfaces we contact [15]. The release of certain chemical agents can be done in ways that make it difficult for victims to identify the fact that they were exposed. However, it is common that chemical agent releases are often characterized by the rapid onset of medical symptoms in humans (minutes to hours), and they may be identified by the presence of a colored residue, dead foliage, pungent odor, and also dead insects and animals.

*The initial clues that a chemical agent was released may be observed as the presence of sick or dying insects, animals, or people at the scene of an emergency event.*

The United States military uses ABC-M8 VGH chemical detector paper as a preliminary means for detecting chemical agents [17]. The M8 paper detects and identifies liquid agents; it does not identify agents in vapor form. The paper comes in booklets of 25 sheets. The papers will identify liquid V or G-type nerve agents or H-type blister agents. The sheets are impregnated with chemical compounds that turn dark green, yellow, or red upon contact with a liquid chemical agent. A color chart in the M8 paper booklet helps to determine the type of agent contacted. The paper when wet by a liquid chemical agent will provide a color indication [17]. In addition, the military uses the M9 chemical agent detector paper as a gross means of detecting G and V agents and/or H and L agents. This paper turns a red color if it contacts any of the above liquid chemical agents [17]. These materials are relatively inexpensive and should be considered for use by first responders.

The following tables detail common chemical agent threats:

Chemical Agent Reference Charts [5]

Nerve Agents [5]

| Common Name (Military Symbol) | Tabun (GA) | Sarin (GB) | Soman (GD) | VX |
|---|---|---|---|---|
| Volatility/ Persistency | Semi-persistent | | | Persistent |
| Rate of Action | Rapid | | | |
| Route of Entry | Respiratory and Skin | | | |
| Odor | Fruity | | Camphor | Sulfur |
| Signs/Symptoms | Headache, runny nose, salivation, pin-point pupils, difficulty in breathing tightness in chest, seizures/convulsions | | | |
| Self-Protection | Respiratory and skin | | | |
| First Aid | Remove from contaminated area, treat symptoms–Atropine and 2-Pam chloride | | | |
| Human Decontamination | Remove agent from skin Flush with warm water/soap | | | |
| Non-persistent agent, dissipates in minutes to hours Semi-persistent agent, dissipates in less than 12 hours Persistent agent, dissipates over time greater than 12 hours | | | | |

## Blister Agents/Vesicants [5]

| Common Name (Military Symbol) | Mustard (H) | Lewisite (L) | Phosgene Oxime (CX) |
|---|---|---|---|
| Volatility/ Persistency | Persistent | | |
| Rate of Action | Delayed | Rapid | |
| Route of Entry | Skin, inhalation, eyes | | |
| Odor | Garlic | Geraniums | Irritating |
| Signs/Symptoms | Red, burning skin, blisters, sore throat, dry cough. Pulmonary edema, memory loss, coma/seizures. *Some symptoms may be delayed from 2 to 24 hours.* | | |
| Self-Protection | Respiratory and skin | | |
| First Aid | Decontaminate with copious amounts of water, remove clothing, support airway, treat symptomatically | | |
| Human Decontamination | Remove agent from skin and flush with warm water and soap | | |
| Non-persistent agent, dissipates in minutes to hours<br>Semi-persistent agent, dissipates in less than 12 hours<br>Persistent agent, dissipates over time greater than 12 hours | | | |

## Blood Agents [5]

| Common Name (Military Symbol) | Hydrogen Cyanide (AC) | Cyanogen Chloride (CK) | Arsine (SA) |
|---|---|---|---|
| Volatility/ Persistency | Non-persistent | | |
| Rate of Action | Rapid | | |
| Route of Entry | Inhalation, skin, and eyes | | |
| Odor | Burnt almonds or peach kernels | | Garlic |
| Signs/Symptoms | Cherry read skin/lips, rapid breathing, dizziness, nausea, vomiting, convulsions, dilated pupils, excessive salivation, gastrointestinal hemorrhage, pulmonary edema, convulsions, respiratory arrest | | |
| Self-Protection | Respiratory and skin | | |
| First Aid | Remove from contaminated area, assist ventilations, treat symptomatically, administer cyanide kit. | | |
| Human Decontamination | Remove contamination from skin, remove wet clothing, flush with soap and water, aerate | | |
| Non-persistent agent, dissipates in minutes to hours<br>Semi-persistent agent, dissipates in less than 12 hours<br>Persistent agent, dissipates over time greater than 12 hours | | | |

Choking Agents [5]

| Common Name (Military Symbol) | Chlorine (CL) | Phosgene (CG) | Diphosgene (DP) |
|---|---|---|---|
| Volatility/ Persistency | Non-persistent Vapors may hang in low areas | | |
| Rate of Action | Rapid in high concentrations Up to 3 hours in low concentrations | | |
| Route of Entry | Respiratory and skin | | |
| Odor | Bleach | Newly mown hay | Cut grass or green corn |
| Signs/Symptoms | Eye and airway irritation, dizziness, tightness in chest, pulmonary edema, painful cough, nausea, headache | | |
| Self-Protection | Respiratory and skin | | |
| First Aid | Remove from contaminated area, remove contaminated clothing, assist ventilations, rest | | |
| Human Decontamination | Wash with copious amounts of water, aerate | | |
| Non-persistent agent, dissipates in minutes to hours Semi-persistent agent, dissipates in less than 12 hours Persistent agent, dissipates over time greater than 12 hours | | | |

## 1.0 DECONTAMINATION FOR CHEMICAL EXPOSURES

Four basic classes of chemical warfare agents are addressed in the tables above. These agent classes are nerve agents, blister/vesicant agents, blood agents, and choking agents. These classes of agents may contain materials specifically produced as chemical warfare agents or may contain materials that are toxic industrial chemicals. Each of these classes of toxic chemicals generally respond well to similar decontamination methods. There are two basic processes used for chemical agent decontamination, physical removal and chemical deactivation. These methods may be used independently or combined to obtain greater efficiency. Each of these decontamination methods and combined methods are described in the following sections [1].

Decontamination by Physical Removal

A significant advantage of physical removal methods is that they generally work well for decontaminating objects that have been exposed to almost any chemical agent. Therefore, knowledge of the specific contamination agent or agents is not required [1]. In addition, normal physical removal methods are not complicated and usually don't require specialized equipment.

Removal of Clothing

Victims who may have been contaminated may have chemical agent liquid on their clothing and skin. Immediate decontamination is essential to prevent or minimize the amount of liquid absorbed in the body.

The removal of a victim's clothing could significantly remove most of the contaminant. It is often cited that removing a victim's clothes could remove about 80% of the contamination [11]. This estimate of course is influenced by what the person is wearing (e.g., a long or short-sleeved shirt, long or short pants, socks and shoes, undershirt, and underwear.)

It has been calculated that if a contaminated person was wearing one of the combinations of clothes listed below, simply removing the clothes would possibly result in the removal of surface contamination in the approximate percentages indicated below:

| | |
|---|---|
| Long-sleeved shirt, long pants, socks, and shoes | 80 % |
| Short-sleeved shirt, long pants, socks, and shoes | 70 % |
| Long-sleeved blouse, skirt, socks, and shoes | 65 % |
| Short-sleeved shirt, short pants, socks, and shoes | 50 % |
| Short-sleeved blouse, skirt, socks, and shoes | 50 % |

The victims should begin removing their clothing from top to the bottom. This should reduce the risk of victims inhaling vapors possibly released due to "off-gassing" or from the liquid in their clothing. If clothing is not removed, the time duration for flushing with water should be at least twice as long as if the clothes are removed.

Note: *If victims refuse to remove all of their clothing, they should be encouraged to remove their clothing at least to their underwear. Personal privacy must be respected; however, every attempt must be made to save lives in these situations.*

Physical Removal by Flushing with Water

In general, physical removal is accomplished using detergents (surfactants) in water combined with physical scrubbing using soft brushes only on protective clothing and equipment. This process will remove most forms of surface contamination including dusts, organic chemicals, and inorganic chemicals [18]. However, this method may not be completely effective for removing oily or tacky organic substances.

Both fresh water and sea water may be used to remove chemical agents. The dominate effect of water and detergent/water solutions in decontamination is the physical removal or dilution of chemical warfare agents. A minor added effect from flushing with water comes from slow hydrolysis (a chemical reaction that degrades chemical agents by forming new less harmful substances), which will help to degrade some chemical agents [1].

Warning: *When decontaminating equipment or humans by flushing with water, do not use high pressure flow systems. Water pressure has been found to force chemical agents into materials and has pushed chemical agents into hair follicles and sweat glands [19].*

Low pressure, high volume water flow is needed to dilute and wash away chemical agents if water is the only process being used for decontamination.

Physical Removal with Absorbent Materials

An example of an absorbent material is the activated charcoal particles used to produce safe breathing air in chemical protective masks. This and similar absorbent materials can be purchased for use in chemical decontamination. However, there are several common materials that may be used to absorb chemical warfare agents. In emergency situations, dry powders such as soap powder, earth or dirt, and flour may be used as an absorbent [1]. In cases of skin contamination, flour application followed by wiping with a wet tissue paper is reported to be effective in removing the nerve agents Soman (GD), VX, and mustard [1][20].

Physical Removal by Wiping or Blotting

When other means of physical removal are not immediately available, wiping or blotting chemical agents to remove them from equipment or human skin can be effective. This results in the direct removal of the agent from the equipment or the skin and will reduce the resultant exposure [19]. Also, wiping or blotting may be required if contamination occurs from an agent that has been thickened to impede the decontamination process. Wiping or blotting motions must be performed carefully to remove the agent. Agents must not be spread or smeared since it will likely result in a greater threat. Wiping and blotting motions should be similar to a person carefully removing ketchup that has dropped on a silk tie.

Experiments have shown that wiping a contaminated area with wet tissues to remove the chemical agent can significantly decrease the absorption of Sarin (GB) into the body [19]. However, smearing or spreading an agent over a larger surface area enhances chemical agent absorption.

Decontamination by Chemical Methods – Oxidation and Hydrolysis

The most important category of chemical decontamination reactions is oxidation using "active chlorine" chemicals like hypochlorite that is contained in common household bleach [1]. In addition, hypochlorite is effective for detoxifying chemical agents by the process of hydrolysis. Hypochlorite solutions act universally against the organophosphorous and mustard agents [1] [9]. These alkaline solutions are typically more effective for inactivating chemical warfare agents than acid solutions. Both VX and HD agents contain sulfur that is readily oxidized by hypochlorite, and the higher pH hypochlorite solutions, pH 8 or higher, successfully detoxifies G agents by hydrolysis [1] [10] [21]. *NFPA 1851, Standard on Selection, Care, and Maintenance of Structural Fire Fighting Protective Ensembles [3] states that normal cleaning and decontamination solutions should have a pH range of 6.0 to 10.5. This indicates that protective fire fighting ensembles should be easily detoxified without damage to the materials when exposed to normal cleaning solutions with a pH of 8 to 10.5.* The pH of the decontamination solution is important in determining the amount of active chlorine concentration available for decontamination. The rate of detoxification increases sharply at pH values higher than 8 and increases by a factor of four for every 18 °F (10 °C) rise in temperature for the cleaning solution [9] [10].

Warning: *High pH alkaline solutions may be harmful to human skin. Precautions must be taken to prevent injury caused by exposure to high pH chemical solutions. Read product labels for first aid instructions.*

Current doctrine in the United States (public health and military applications) specify the use of a 0.5 % sodium hypochlorite or calcium hypochlorite solution for decontamination of the skin and a 5 % solution for decontamination of equipment [1]. Household laundry bleach containing sodium hypochlorite and/or calcium hypochlorite is easily found in grocery stores and industrial cleaning supply stores.

Many common household laundry detergents also have high pH alkaline concentrations that would be effective for detoxifying protective clothing materials. pH levels for these detergents may be determined by contacting the manufacturer or by mixing a detergent solution and measuring the pH.

Preliminary Decontamination for Chemical Agent Exposures

The procedure listed in this section is a modification of the Level C Extreme Hazard procedure presented in the NFPA, Hazardous Materials Response Handbook [6].

Important Note: *Much of the decontamination process is done while the first responder is actively using their SCBA. Efforts must be made to provide change-out capability for air cylinders or fixed airline supply for personnel while they are undergoing decontamination. The person doing the decontamination and cylinder exchange must wear protective clothing, gauntlet type butyl rubber gloves, and SCBA [22]. Care must be taken with gauntlet gloves to prevent contaminated materials from flowing down into the glove from the top. Medical gloves may be used inside of gauntlet gloves, and taping may help to prevent contamination from contacting the hands. If Environmental Protection Agency (EPA) "Level B" disposable chemical garments are available, they should be worn.[22].*

Decontamination Procedure:

The decontamination procedures presented provide the basic information for decontaminating first responders at the scene of a chemical agent incident. Incident Commanders may alter these procedures if conditions require changes.

1. A decontamination crew is assembled. It dons protective clothing, SCBAs, and lays out the decontamination areas and corridor.

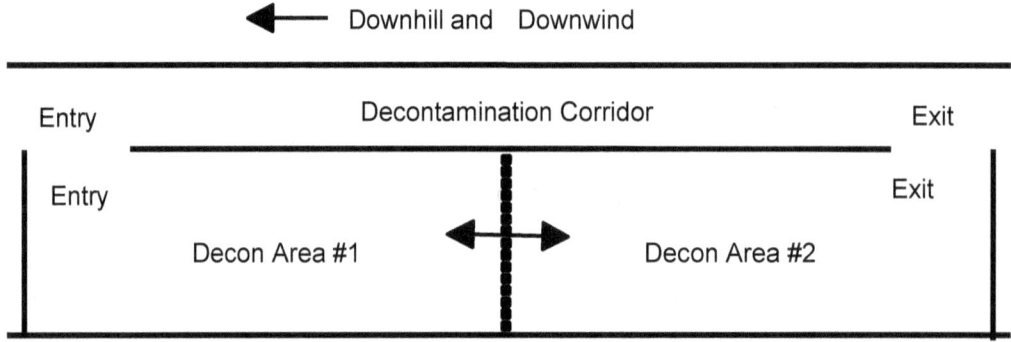

Figure 1. Decontamination Area Layout

32

2.  The crew lays water supply lines needed for decontamination, and prepares a supply of detergent and water solution in a large clean container.  Large soft scrub brushes will be positioned in the decontamination area.  If a soap detergent solution and brushes are not available use large volumes of low-pressure water for decontamination.  *Do not use brushes to scrub human skin.*

3.  The decontamination crew begins decontamination triage as first responders return from work.

Decontamination Triage:

1.  Evaluate personnel for signs of chemical agent toxicity, skin, and protective equipment contamination.  Decontaminate personnel exhibiting the need for medical attention first.

2.  If no personnel show signs of chemical agent toxicity, but have indications that a chemical agent has contacted the skin or hair then decontaminate those personnel next.  It should be remembered that personnel with physically damaged (cut or torn) PPE may be receiving a higher dose of chemical agent than someone with fully intact gear.

3.  If no personnel have indications of chemical agent exposure to the skin or hair, then decontaminate the person having the greatest amount of chemical agent showing on their PPE and work down to the individual having the smallest amount of visible agent.

4.  If no personnel have chemical agent contamination showing on their PPE, then decontaminate the first responder with the lowest air supply first.  Be sure to decontaminate all personnel leaving the hot zone to insure that the chemical agent is not spread to safe areas.

Decontamination Process:

Warning:    *No one involved in the decontamination process, either personnel being decontaminated or personnel doing the decontamination work, should eat, drink, or smoke while in the decontamination area.  All personnel must be careful not to touch the face or other skin surfaces with contaminated hands, gloves, or other contaminated materials during the decontamination process.*

1.  The contaminated first responder will enter decontamination area #1.  (Figure 1)

2.  Do not remove the SCBA facepiece.  The SCBA will be used throughout the decontamination process to supply safe, clean air to the individual undergoing decontamination.

3.  Place the helmet on the back of the neck, suspended by the neck strap.  If you desire to remove the helmet, decontaminate it by flushing with water, remove it, flush the interior, and then place the helmet in an area set aside for decontaminated equipment.

4. If the air supply must be changed during the decontamination process, the mask, associated regulator, hoses, and valves must be thoroughly flushed before changing the air supply. First responders while still wearing the mask must hold their breath while the change-out is in progress. Be careful not to break the mask seal. When the change-out is completed, exhale part of the breath to purge the mask and carefully inhale to insure that the system is working properly before taking a full breath.

5. Flush in sequence downwards from head to toe with copious amounts of low pressure water. Using a soft brush, brush with detergent solution if available. Flush the inside and outside of the helmet, hood if worn, all outside surfaces of the mask, SCBA cylinder, harness, hoses, valves, outside coat surfaces, outside surfaces (including surface folds) of coat wrist cuffs, gloves, bunker pants, and boots.

6. Tools carried by first responders must also be flushed with water and washed to remove contamination.

7. When all visible contamination has been removed, the first responder will advance to decontamination area #2 (Figure 1) and remove their protective clothing and equipment.

Doff and Securing Decontaminated PPE:

1. Remove helmet.

2. Remove gloves.

3. Remove the air supply connection (regulator) from the SCBA mask, and doff the SCBA tank and harness. If the cylinder, harness, hoses, and valves were contaminated, place these items in thick walled, 6 mil (0.15 mm) or thicker, garbage bags and seal the bags for return to the station or other location for decontamination. Label the bags to indicate the contents.

4. Remove the hood, if worn.

5. Remove the SCBA mask.

6. Remove the turnout coat.

7. Remove boots.

8. Remove bunker pants.

9. Disposable over boots may be used to cover the feet until proper footwear is obtained.

10. If circumstances permit, bag all additional protective clothing and equipment that were contaminated. Place items in thick walled,

6 mil (0.15 mm) or thicker, garbage bags and seal the bags for return to the station.  Label the bags with the person's name and the contents of the bag.

Emergency Field Decontamination of Equipment

In the event that an apparatus crew must be immediately dispatched to a following incident, additional measures must be taken to insure that their personal protective clothing and equipment have been decontaminated.  In this situation, all gear should be washed down with one of the detoxification solutions listed in Section I - 3.2 starting on page 10 and discussed in the Section III, page 31, entitled, Decontamination by Chemical Methods – Oxidation and Hydrolysis.  The chlorite-based chemical solutions and high alkaline pH solutions are suitable for the decontamination process.  Rugged plastic pump sprayers used for gardening are considered suitable for dispensing decontamination solutions.  After the decontamination chemicals have been applied and allowed to stay in place for the specified time, the equipment should be thoroughly flushed with water.

Note: *It is important to remember that some decontamination solutions may cause a level of deterioration in the protective equipment.  See Section I – 4.0, page 16.*

Post Doffing Evaluation:

When all gear has been removed, each first responder must be checked to insure that the chemical agent did not contact the skin or hair.  If it is found that the person has chemical agent contamination, immediately do the following:

1. Blot any excess chemical agent from the skin.  Be sure to secure all materials used for blotting agents.  They are still a threat.

2. Strip from the body any additional clothing that may be contaminated.

3. Flush the body with copious amounts of water.  Soap and water is better.  Check to be sure decontamination is complete.

4. Cover the victim to prevent chill and further loss of body heat.

5. Provide immediate medical care.

Final Step:  When all personnel have been successfully decontaminated, the decontamination crew will decontaminate each other following the steps above.

Actions Upon Returning to the Station

1. Secure apparatus on the exterior of station.

2. Secure all contaminated materials in an exterior cordoned-off area away from public access.

Personal hygiene:

3. Strip completely and place all clothing, protective and personal, in plastic bags. Seal and label the bags. Place bags in exterior cordoned-off area.

4. Shower and shampoo hair. Wash in sequence from head to toe scrubbing all of the body with soap and water. Care should be taken to insure that areas around the mouth (mustache), nostrils, under fingernails, under arms, and groin areas are clean.

Note: *Research of fire fighters using turnout gear in simulated chemical weapons agent environments showed that moist areas of the body (e.g. groin and under arms) are most susceptible to some chemical agents [23].*

5. Personnel exposed to chemical agents should receive a medical examination.

# Section IV

# BIOLOGICAL WARFARE INCIDENTS

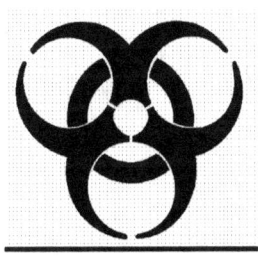

*Biological Agent Symbol*

## IV. BIOLOGICAL AGENT EXPOSURES

Biological agents can be dispersed in the air we breath, in the water we drink, or on surfaces we contact [15]. The release of biological agents can be done in ways that make it difficult for victims to identify the fact that they were exposed. The first indication of a biological attack may occur hours or days after victims were exposed to an agent. *The initial clues that a biological agent was released may result from an unusual number of sick or dying animals, or people in a community.* By the time that it is confirmed that a biological attack has occurred, many first responders and their equipment may have already been exposed to the threat. In this case, efforts must be made to provide preventive medical treatment for all of the exposed first responders, and immediate action is needed to decontaminate all exposed personnel and their emergency equipment.

Biological Agent Reference Chart [5]

| Agent | Dissemination | Transmission (person to person) | Incubation | Lethality |
|---|---|---|---|---|
| Anthrax | Spores in aerosol | No (except cutaneous) | 1 to 5 days | High |
| Botulinum Toxin | Ingestion and aerosol | No | Hours to days | High |
| Ricin | Ingestion and aerosol | No | Hours to days | High |
| Plague | Aerosol | High | 1 to 3 days | High if untreated |
| Ebola | Contact and aerosol | Moderate | 4 to 16 days | Moderate to high |
| T-2 Mycotoxins | Ingestion and aerosol | No | 2 to 4 days | Moderate |
| Tularemia (Rabbit fever) | Aerosol | No | 1 to 10 days | Moderate if untreated |
| Cholera | Ingestion and aerosol | Rare | 12 hours to 6 days | Low with treatment |
| Smallpox | Aerosol | High | 10 to 12 days | Low |
| VEE | Aerosol and infected vectors | Low | 1 to 6 days | Low |
| Q Fever | Ingestion and aerosol | Rare | 14 to 16 days | Very low |
| Staphylococal Enterotoxin | Ingestion and aerosol | No | Hours | less than 1 % |

## 1.0 DECONTAMINATION FOR BIOLOGICAL EXPOSURES

The procedure listed in this section is a modification of the Level C Extreme Hazard procedure presented in the NFPA, Hazardous Materials Response Handbook [6].

Important Note: *Much of the decontamination process is done while the first responder is actively using their SCBA. Efforts must be made to provide change-out capability for air cylinders or fixed hose air supply for personnel while they are undergoing decontamination.*

*The person doing the decontamination and cylinder exchange must wear protective clothing, including protective gloves, and SCBA or other suitable respiratory mask.*
*If EPA "Level B" disposable chemical garments are available, they should be worn.[22].*

Decontamination Procedure:

The decontamination procedures presented provide the basic information for decontaminating first responders at the scene of a biological agent incident. Incident commanders may alter these procedures if conditions require changes.

1. A decontamination crew is assembled. It lays out the decontamination areas and corridor, and begins decontamination triage as first responders return from work.

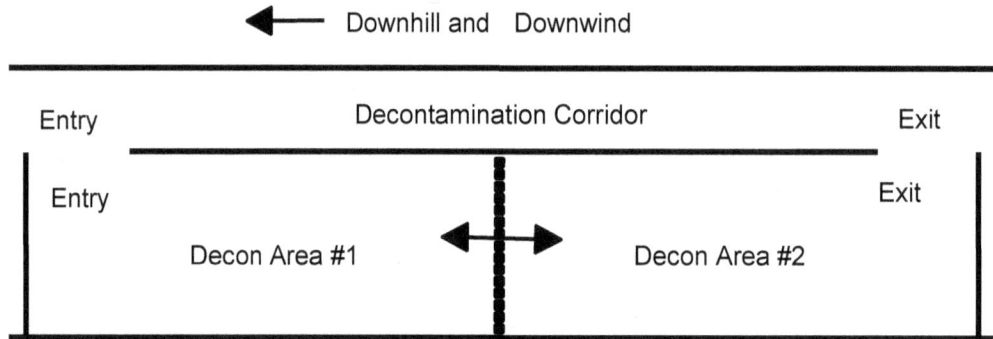

Figure 1. Decontamination Area Layout

Decontamination Triage:

1. Evaluate personnel for signs of agent toxicity, skin, and protective equipment contamination. Decontaminate personnel exhibiting the need for medical attention first.

2. If no personnel exhibit signs of agent toxicity, but have indications that a biological agent has contacted the skin or hair decontaminate those personnel next. It should be remembered that personnel with physically damaged (cut or torn) PPE are more likely to have skin contamination from biological agents.

3. If no personnel show indications that their body was contaminated by a suspected biological agent, then decontaminate the person having the greatest amount of suspected agent showing on their PPE and work down to the individual having the smallest amount of visible agent.

4. If no personnel have suspected biological agent contamination showing on their PPE, then decontaminate the first responder with the lowest air reserve first. Be sure to decontaminate all personnel leaving the hot zone to insure that the biological agent is not spread to safe areas.

Decontamination Process:

Warning :   *No one involved in the decontamination process either personnel being decontaminated or personnel doing the decontamination work should eat, drink, or smoke while in the decontamination area.  All personnel must be careful not to touch the face or other skin surfaces with contaminated hands, gloves, or other contaminated materials during the decontamination process.*

1.  The contaminated first responder will enter decontamination area #1.

2.  Do not remove the SCBA facepiece.  The SCBA will be used throughout the decontamination process to supply safe clean air to the individual undergoing decontamination.

3.  Place the helmet on the back of the neck, suspended by the neck strap.

4.  If the air supply must be changed during the decontamination process, the mask, associated regulator, hoses, and valves must be thoroughly flushed before changing the air supply.  First responders, while still wearing the mask, must hold their breath while the change-out is in progress.  Be careful not to break the mask seal.  When the change-out is completed, exhale part of the breath to purge the mask and carefully inhale to insure that the system is working properly before taking a full breath.

5.  Flush first responder downwards from head to toe with copious amounts of low pressure water.  Flush the inside and outside of the helmet, hood if worn, all outside surfaces of the mask, SCBA cylinder, harness, hoses, valves, outside coat surfaces, outside surfaces (including surface folds) of coat wrist cuffs, gloves, bunker pants, and boots.

6.  Tools carried by first responders must also be flushed with water to remove contamination.

7.  When all visible contamination has been removed, the first responder will advance to decontamination area #2 and remove their protective clothing and equipment.

Doff and Securing Decontaminated PPE:

       1.  Remove helmet.

       2.  Remove gloves.

       3.  Remove the air supply connection (regulator) from the SCBA mask, and doff the SCBA tank and harness.  If the cylinder, harness, hoses, and valves were contaminated, place these items in thick walled, 6 mil (0.15 mm) or thicker, garbage bags and seal the bags for return to the station.  Label the bags to indicate the contents.

4. Remove the hood, if worn.

5. Remove the SCBA mask

6. Remove the turnout coat

7. Remove boots.

8. Remove bunker pants.

9. If circumstances permit, bag all additional protective clothing and equipment that were contaminated. Place items in thick walled, 6 mil (0.15 mm) or thicker, garbage bags and seal the bags for return to the station. Label the bags with the person's name and the contents of the bag.

Emergency Field Decontamination of Equipment

In the event that an apparatus crew must be immediately dispatched to another incident, additional measures must be taken to insure that their personal protective clothing and equipment have been decontaminated. In this situation, all gear should be washed down with one of the detoxification solutions listed in Section I - 3.2, page 10 and discussed in Section III, page 31, entitled, Decontamination by Chemical Methods – Oxidation and Hydrolysis. The chlorite based chemical solutions are suitable for the decontamination process. Rugged plastic pump sprayers used for gardening have been found to be suitable for dispensing decontamination solutions. After the decontamination chemicals have been applied and allowed to stay in place for the specified time, the equipment should be thoroughly flushed with water.

Note: *It is important to remember that some decontamination solutions may cause a level of deterioration in the protective equipment.*

Post Doffing Evaluation:

When all gear has been removed, each first responder must be checked to insure that the biological agents did not contact the skin or hair. If it is found that a person has been contamination by a potential biological agent, do the following:

1. Gently wet any suspected biological agent concentrations on the skin and/or personal clothing. This helps to prevent the agent from becoming airborne and reduces the chances that the agent will be inhaled.

2. Strip any additional clothing from the body that may be contaminated.

3. Flush the body with copious amounts of water. Soap and water is better.

4. Cover the victim to prevent chill and further loss of body heat.

5. Provide immediate medical care, if needed.

Final Step: When all personnel have been successfully decontaminated, the decontamination crew will decontaminate each other following the steps above.

Actions Upon Returning to the Station

> 1. Secure apparatus on the exterior of station.
>
> 2. Secure all contaminated materials in an exterior cordoned-off area away from public access.
>
> Personal hygiene:
>
> 3. Strip completely and place all clothing, protective and personal, in plastic bags. Seal and label the bags. Place bags in exterior cordoned-off area.
>
> 4. Shower. Shampoo hair. Wash in sequence from head to toe scrubbing all of the body with soap and water. Care should be taken to insure that areas around the mouth (mustache), nostrils, under fingernails, under arms, and groin areas are clean.
>
> 5. Personnel exposed to potential biological agents should receive follow-up medical care.

## CHEMICAL METHODS FOR BIOLOGICAL WARFARE AGENT DECONTAMINATION.

The most often recommended method for decontamination of materials exposed to biological agents using chemical methods is associated with the use of chlorine containing solutions. Manufacturers of fibers and fabric materials used in the manufacturer of fire service protective clothing materials do not recommend that their materials be exposed to laundry detergents, bleaches, or disinfectants containing chlorine. Particularly, fabrics containing Kevlar® fibers are susceptible to loss of strength after exposure to chlorine. However, laboratory tests have shown that a single short time exposure to a common commercial household chlorine bleach (6 % sodium hypochlorite solution) will not seriously degrade fabrics containing Kevlar®, and it will decontaminate garments exposed to all known biological agents. Therefore, the following procedure may be used in emergency situations to decontaminate fire service PPE using a commercial household chlorine bleach solution [24][25]:

# EMERGENCY DECONTAMINATION USING POOL AND SPA SANITIZERS

The following 68 % available chlorine calcium hypochlorite solutions are suggested formulations that may be used for decontaminating CWA and BWA agents [11]:

Warning: *No information is available on the potential harmful effects that pool and spa sanitizing solutions may have on first responders' personal protective clothing and equipment. To determine the potential for damage, pretest solutions on old gear that is being decommissioned.*

Note: *A contact time of 15 minutes is recommended for use against all biological agents, including spores [11].*

Personnel decontamination [11]: 0.5 % solution for CWA and BWA. Add 0.5 lb (227 g) of HTH to 12 gal of water and carefully mix until completely blended.

Equipment decontamination [11]: 2 % solution for BWA. Add 1 lb (454 g) of HTH to 6 gal of water and carefully mix until completely blended.

# EMERGENCY DECONTAMINATION USING 6 % CHLORINE BLEACH

Warning : *This treatment is for emergency decontamination only and should be used only one time on materials containing Kevlar®. See Section 4, page 16.*

- Completely soak the protective clothing and equipment for one minute in undiluted Ultra Clorox® regular bleach or an equivalent product that contains a 6 % sodium hypochlorite solution.
- Do not dilute the manufacturer's bleach solution with water, as is normally done.
- After the one minute soak in the ultra chlorine bleach solution, immediately rinse the protective clothing with large quantities of tepid water. Air dry or use appropriate machine drying processes.

Note: *Some materials may show a change in color.*

Warning : *For Kevlar® containing fabrics, repeated exposures to chlorine containing solutions will result in serious loss of material strength and will cause the protective clothing systems to fail when in normal use. See Section 4.*

Effectiveness: The above decontamination procedure will inactivate 99.8 % of anthrax spores in one minute and will completely inactivate E. coli over the same time period [25].

# NORMAL DECONTAMINATION USING 6 % CHLORINE BLEACH

Use on fire fighters' protective clothing and equipment that does not contain materials that are seriously degraded by exposure to chlorine solutions.

This process may be used on protective equipment that does not contain Kevlar® and has firm or hard equipment surfaces: Examples: helmets, rubber boots, some gloves, SCBA tanks and harness frames, masks, rubber hoses, and external regulator surfaces.

Warning : *Check with your SCBA manufacturer for decontamination procedures for internal components of SCBA regulators and masks.*

- Completely soak the protective clothing and equipment for 15 minutes in a household bleach (sodium hypochlorite) solution that has been diluted to produce a 0.26 % (1:22) bleach solution.
- After the 15 minute soak in the 1:22 bleach solution, immediately rinse the protective clothing and equipment with large quantities of tepid water.

Effectiveness: The above decontamination procedure will inactivate 100 % of anthrax spores exposed to the treatment [25].

## PHYSICAL METHODS FOR BIOLOGICAL WARFARE AGENT DECONTAMINATION

Fire fighters' protective ensembles that meet the requirements of the NFPA 1971 standard [2] must pass a test for "Heat and Thermal Shrinkage Resistance." This test exposes ensemble components to an oven test to determine if the materials will degrade when exposed for five minutes to an oven temperature of 260 °C (500 °F). The test requires that the materials must not ignite, melt, drip, or separate following the exposure. In addition, the materials must not exhibit excessive shrinkage after the exposure. Requirements for this standard, as well as research results from other studies, indicate that the fire fighters' protective ensemble should withstand the dry heat exposures listed below for biological agent decontamination. Since there is no available data on the response of fire fighting ensemble components to steam heat or autoclaving uncertainty exists related to gear performance after the exposure. Research experience at NIST and discussions with equipment manufacturers indicate that most components of NFPA 1971 compliant fire fighting ensembles will withstand the exposure to a steam heat decontamination procedure without performance changes. However, it is cautioned that some moisture barrier materials may experience a level of degradation as a result of exposure to a steam heat decontamination process.

DRY HEAT METHOD:

Expose biologically contaminated materials to one of the following temperature/time conditions [1][26]:

*180 °C (356 °F) for ................30 minutes*
*170 °C (340 °F) for .............1 hour*
*160 °C (320 °F) for............... 2 hours*
*150 °C (300 °F) for .............2.5 hours*

Some fire training facilities have live fire training compartments that may be adapted for the above dry heat method of decontamination. It is critical that all components and parts of the materials being decontaminated reach the recommended dry heat temperature, and they must be maintained at the given temperature for at least the specified time period.

STEAM HEAT METHOD, AUTOCLAVING:

- Expose contaminated materials to a pressure of 1 atmosphere (15 psi or 103 kPa) above normal atmospheric pressure with a steam temperature of 121 °C (250 °F) and a decontamination exposure time of 20 minutes [26].

No field expedient method has been identified to replicate the steam heat method. However, many medical and some research facilities have large autoclaves that could be used for biological agent decontamination.

# Section V

# RADIOLOGICAL MATERIALS IONIZING RADIATION INCIDENTS

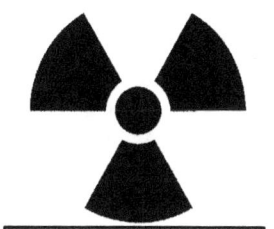

*Radioactive Material Symbol*

## V. RADIOLOGICAL MATERIALS AND IONIZING RADIATION

The possibility of terrorist attacks with nuclear weapons and/or a radiation dispersal device (RDD) has increased as terrorist organizations have advanced in sophistication [27]. As a result, first responders must be able to recognize and safely control scenes where such weapons have been used. The detonation of small nuclear weapons initially may not appear much different from the explosion of a large conventional explosive weapon. Observable physical damage is likely to be similar. However, the nuclear weapon carries with it the possibility of injury from radiological materials. In addition, radiological dispersal devices may use conventional explosives to disperse radiological materials ("dirty bombs") that can cause physical injuries, contamination, and unnecessary panic.

In events where nuclear weapons have been detonated or where radiological materials have been released, *it is critical that emergency first responders have instruments for identifying the presence of the radiological materials*. Radiological materials are relatively easy to identify as compared to biological, and many of the chemical agents that exist, and it doesn't require extensive training to be able to use the more basic radiological detection instruments. *All emergency first response units must have a basic functional means to identify the existence of radiological materials at the scene of a suspected CBRN incident.* Many modern instruments for detecting the presence of radiological materials are relatively inexpensive to buy and are designed for rugged use.

*It is recommended that at least one first responder with each entry team at a possible CBRN incident be fitted with an electronic ionizing radiation dosimeter. This dosimeter should have an audible alarm that is triggered by the presence of radioactive materials. Electronic ionizing radiation dosimeters of this type are small, light weight, and may be easily clipped to the fire fighter's personal protective clothing or equipment. In addition, each fire apparatus should have a high range radioactive materials detection instrument that is capable of measuring ionizing radiation exposures over the range of at least 1 R/hr to 50 R/hr.*

## THREATS FROM IONIZING RADIATION

There are four primary exposure threats from nuclear radiation. They are: alpha particles, beta particles, gamma rays, and neutrons. All four are immediately released at the instant a fission weapon (atomic weapon) is detonated. However, there is no residual threat from neutrons since they are released at the instant the explosion occurs. Materials emitting ionizing radiation, alpha particles, beta particles, and gamma rays are expected to be persistent after the WMD has been detonated. With a "dirty bomb" or other types of RDDs, there will generally be no threat from neutrons since neutrons are not emitted during the discharge of a RDD, and common radiological materials do not normally emit neutrons.

Alpha Particles [28]

Alpha particles lose energy rapidly in matter and do not penetrate very far; however, they can cause damage over their short path through tissue. These particles are usually completely absorbed by the outer dead layer of the human skin, so, alpha emitting radioisotopes are not a hazard outside the body. However, materials that emit alpha particles can be very harmful if they are ingested, inhaled, or enter the body through openings in the human skin. Alpha particles can be stopped completely by a sheet of paper.

Beta Particles [28]

Beta particles are fast moving and are more penetrating than alpha particles, but are less damaging over equally traveled distances. Some beta particles are capable of penetrating human skin and cause radiation damage; however, as with alpha emitters, materials that emit beta particles are generally more hazardous when they are inhaled, ingested, or enter the body through openings in the human skin. Beta particles travel a few meters in air, but can be reduced or stopped by 2 to 3 layers of clothing, turnout gear, or by a few millimeters of a material such as aluminum. If materials emitting beta particles are on the skin inside of clothing, they will likely cause injury to the skin.

Note: *Standard fire fighters' turnout gear will protect a person from external alpha and beta nuclear radiation hazards. Beta radiation is considered to be an external health threat to the skin and eyes.*

Gamma Rays [28]

Gamma rays are much like X-rays in that they travel at the speed of light and are very penetrating. Gamma rays can easily pass completely through the human body or be absorbed by the tissue. This causes a serious radiation hazard for the entire body and causes severe damage to internal organs. Several feet of concrete or a few inches of lead may be required to stop the penetration of gamma rays.

The following diagram exhibits the ability of ionizing radiation to penetrate matter [27]:

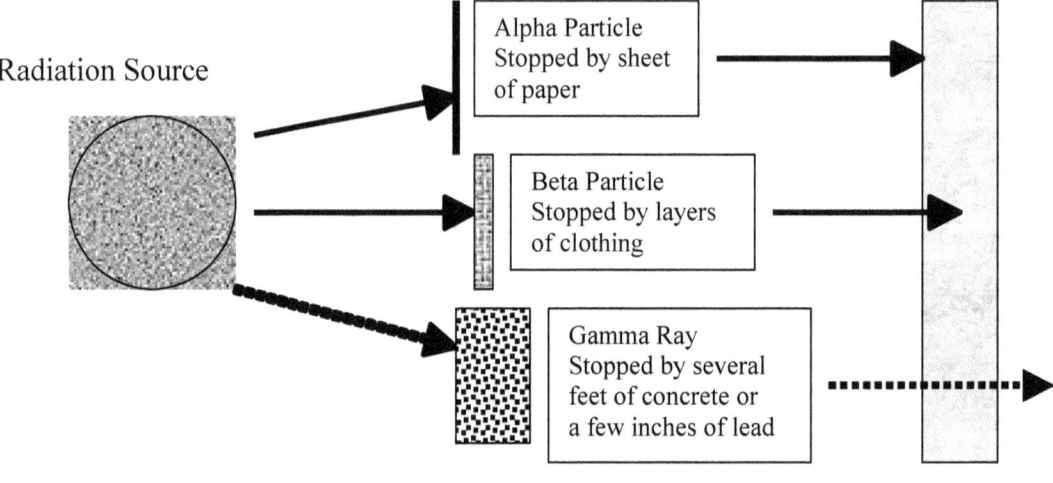

Figure A. Penetrating ability of nuclear radiation.

Neutrons [28]

Neutrons can travel long distances in air and are released during nuclear fission. (Nuclear fission occurs during nuclear reactor operations or the explosion of an atomic bomb.) Like gamma rays, neutrons present an extreme hazard for human exposure. Water, concrete, or any material with a high hydrogen content offers the best shielding from neutrons. Neutrons may be encountered where nuclear fuels are undergoing fission. This should be expected around nuclear reactors or with a WMD that produces a nuclear reaction.

## PERSONAL RADIATION DETECTOR

The following personal radiation detection and alarm instrument used by the United States Military may be useful for fire service operations. It is small, relatively light weight "about 10 oz (284 g)", and rugged [29].

*UDR-13 or UDR-13A, Radiac Set, portable radiation detector for Neutron/Gamma radiation dose and Gamma dose rate. The unit is powered by four AAA batteries and operates in the normal mode for about 100 hours. The units are capable of measuring and displaying (13 Radiac, 1 mR/h to 999 R/h)(13A Radiac, 1 μR/h to 300 R/h) gamma radiation dose rate. The dosimeter module is capable of measuring, storing and displaying dose from 1 μR to 999 R. The instrument also incorporates a presettable alarm and a sleep mode. The sleep mode allows for automatic, periodic, short-time displays of dose rate, and operating time in the sleep mode will extend operational time to about 290 hours. The instrument also comes with a carrying case with a clip for attaching it to a belt or harness. The instrument measures 3.9 in x 2.6 in x 1 in (100 mm x 65 mm x 25 mm). Unit price is about $800. Additional information available by contacting Canberra Dover (formally Aptec-NRC), 58 Richboynton Road, Dover, New Jersey 07801 [29].*

## SURFACE RADIATION CONTAMINATION MONITOR

There are a number of hand held detectors on the market that can be used as a radiation surface contamination measurement device. These instruments may be used as a low-level contamination survey instrument. They may also be used to determine if fire and rescue personnel and their equipment have been contaminated by radioactive materials. The instruments are also useful for measuring the effectiveness of decontamination procedures. The basic contamination monitor is a small hand held design incorporating a "pancake GM tube" (GM, Geiger-Mueller sensor) detector. This detector will detect the presence of beta and gamma radiation. Small, rugged instruments are manufactured by several companies. The cost of the instrument is approximately $500. The following is an example of an instrument suitable for contamination monitoring [30]:

*Model No. TBM-3SR is a rugged metal cased model with an analog meter having three "count per minute" (cpm) output ranges. The ranges are 0 to 500, 0 to 5000, 0 to 50,000 cpm. The cpm scale is most useful for decontamination measurements. The meter also has a mR/h scale. The instrument has an audio alert the gives an audible indication of count change. Physical dimensions for the unit are: 3 in x 5.25 in x 2.25 in (76 mm x 133 mm x 60 mm) excluding the removable handle height. The instrument weighs 22 oz (625 g). Electrical power is supplied by a standard 9 volt battery that will operate the unit for approximately 100 hours. . The instrument is manufactured by Technical Associates, 7051 Eton Avenue, Canoga Park, CA 91303 [30].*

Many radiation monitor manufacturers will sell a safe low-level radiation check source for checking an instrument's operation. However, potassium chloride ("Nu-Salt" or an equivalent salt substitute) may be used to easily check the operation of a radiation detection meter. The potassium chloride should only be used to check the operation of thin-walled pancake GM tubes. It will not work successfully with thick-walled GM tubes or with gamma detectors. The meter should be turned on and set to the x1 scale. The normal background counts per minute (cpm) should be very low. Pour some potassium chloride salt on a flat surface and place the instrument close to and directly above the sample. The meter needle should rise above the normal background level and provide a reading of 100 to 200 (cpm) or more. This reading will demonstrate that the meter is operating. The salt substitute can be purchased in most grocery stores. The potassium chloride produces a very low and harmless level of radiation. However, it is adequate to increase measurement levels above normal background radiation levels and provides a safe check for instrument operation. Additional emitters of natural radiation are luminescent dials and gauges, some ceramic ware (fiestaware), and some Coleman lantern mantles.

Health Effects of Ionizing Radiation [27][15]

During attacks using nuclear devices or radiation dispersal devices, it is expected that people will be exposed to dangerous levels of ionizing radiation. Threats to human health from ionizing radiation are well known, and the pathways for these radiological exposures are well defined.

Exposure pathways listed in the table below must be considered during decontamination:

Table 1. Human Exposure from Radiological Incidents [27] [31]
Possible exposure pathways during a radiological emergency involving a WMD.

| Exposure Pathway | Exposure Source |
|---|---|
| External exposure | Ionizing radiation from detonation of a WMD<br>Exposure to the detonation plume.<br>Exposure to fallout from the plume.<br>Surface contamination and activation products.<br>Personal contamination (skin, hair, and clothing). |
| Internal exposure (contamination) | Inhalation of plume.<br>Inhalation of air suspended contamination.<br>Inhalation or ingestion of personal contamination (radioactive materials on clothing or the human body).<br>Ingestion of contaminated food.<br>Absorption of contaminated material through skin, or injection of contaminated material into the skin (as through a wound). |

If radioactive materials enter the human body, the hazard is much greater than the same exposure to external skin contamination. Trivial levels of radiological materials that contaminate external skin surfaces may become very significant health threats if the same levels of contamination are introduced into the human body [27] [31].

Ionizing radiation as discussed above can cause changes in the chemical balance and function of human cells or kill the cells. Some of those changes can result in cancer or damage to DNA that can cause harmful genetic mutations. Exposure to very large amounts of radiation can cause radiation sickness in a few hours or days and death within 60 days of the exposure. In extreme cases, it can cause death within a few hours of exposure.

The two principal effects of radiation on humans is manifested as: 1) Internal Contamination or 2) Acute Radiation Syndrome (ARS).

Internal contamination occurs when a person ingests, inhales or is wounded by a radioactive material and there is skin absorption. Exposure will continue until the material is flushed from the body. Acute Radiation Syndrome is a sequence of phased clinical syndromes occurring in stages during a period of hours to weeks after an exposure. The time period depends on an individual's radiation sensitivity, type of radiation exposure, and the dose of radiation absorbed. The "Prodromal Phase" is characterized by the onset of nausea, vomiting, and malaise. The time to onset from exposure, in the absence of other associated trauma, is dependent on dose. The "Latent Phase" follows the "Prodromal Phase" and is characterized in the victim by a relatively symptom free period. The length of this phase will again depend on the exposure dose. Following the symptom free period the victim will present with clinical symptoms associated with affected major organ system/systems (bone marrow, gastro-intestinal, cardio-neuro-vascular). There is then either a Recovery Phase or death [15]. Note: *It is unlikely that a radiation dispersal device (RDD) will produce radiation levels high enough to cause acute radiation syndrome except, in close proximity to the source of materials release.*

Radiation Sickness:

*Mild* - a human may experience nausea, mild headache, lack of appetite, and fatigue within a few hours after exposure (threshold >25 R) [27] [32].

*Moderate* - a human may experience skin reddening (due to beta dose), nausea, lack of appetite, and fatigue within 2 to 3 hours of exposure, prostration (physical and mental exhaustion) may occur, symptoms may improve and then reoccur, potential for delayed wound healing (full recovery expected up to 200 R) [27] [32].

*Severe* - a human may experience nausea, lack of appetite, fatigue and prostration which will then clear up. After a week or more, fever, mouth soreness, and diarrhea may appear; gums and mouth ulcerate and bleed; patients may lose hair, and develop increased infection susceptibility, hypotension, and sudden vascular collapse. Some people will die. (250 to 500 R most recover) [27] [32].

The following is a general description of radiation sickness that includes recent findings: For humans, radiation sickness is associated with gastrointestinal disorders, bacterial infections, hemorrhaging, anemia, loss of body fluids, and electrolyte imbalance. Very large doses of radiation can cause extensive cellular damage and result in death. Delayed effects can include cataracts, temporary or permanent sterility, cancer, and genetic effects [27] [31].

Normal background exposure rate for gamma radiation is approximately 0.01 to 0.03 milliroentgen per hour (mR/h) or 10 to 30 microroentgen per hour ( μR/h) on sensitive gamma survey instruments [22]. See Appendix B for radiological unit conversion tables. In emergency situations normal work using fire fighter turnout gear and SCBA can continue with elevated exposure rates; however, if the exposure rate increases 3 to 5 times above normal gamma background, operations should be monitored to insure first responder safety [22]. Radiological monitoring is the responsibility of each first responder, unit officers, and the incident commander. A health physicist should be consulted if an exposure rate of 1 mR/h (0.01 mSv/h.) or above is measured [27]. The National Council on Radiation Protection and Measurements (NCRP) recommends that *an ambient dose rate of approximately 10 mR/h (0.1 mSv/h) is a suitable initial alarm level for radiation detection and alarm instruments* [27]. NCRP also recommends *a second alarm level, the turn around and leave level, to have an ambient dose rate and ambient dose for emergency operations purposes to be approximately 10 R/h or 10 R (0.1 Sv/h or 0.1 Sv).* This second alarm level is recommended to provide the first responder with the capability to work on critical issues of a compelling nature [27]. These critical issues include the rescue of injured persons and time-sensitive actions to gain control of the scene [27]. Also, work activities at higher exposure levels may be possible if managed by a health physicist, and there is appropriate operational equipment available [27]. Note: *The above alarm levels are appropriate for personnel protection from gamma radiation; however, they should not be used for marking contamination zone boundaries.*

Table 2. Whole body radiation dose guidelines for emergency operations and acute health effects [27][33].

| Whole Body Dose Limits rem (Sv) | Work Activity | Work Conditions | Health Effects (without medical treatment) |
|---|---|---|---|
| 0.001 rem (0.01 mSv) | All work activities | Request radiation support personnel. Use personal dosimeters. | None |
| 0.01 rem (0.1 mSv) | All work activities | Initial instrument alarm level | None |
| 5 rem (0.05 Sv) | All work activities | Monitor conditions | None |
| 10 rem (0.1 Sv) | Lifesaving, protection of critical property | Where a lower dose limit is not practical | None |
| 25 rem (0.25 Sv) | Lifesaving or protection of large populations | Where a lower dose limit is not practical | Blood changes, no illness |
| >25 rem (>0.25 Sv) | Lifesaving or protection of large populations | Only on a voluntary basis for personnel fully aware of the risks involved. | Possible radiation sickness, no death |
| 100 rem (1 Sv) | Lifesaving or protection of large populations | Only on a voluntary basis for personnel fully aware of the risks involved | Possible radiation sickness, no death |
| 450 rem (4.5) Sv | - | - | 50 % death rate |
| 1,000 rem (10 Sv) | - | - | 100 % death rate |

## 1.0 DECONTAMINATION FOR RADIOLOGICAL MATERIALS EXPOSURES

Preliminary Decontamination for Radiological Materials Exposures

The procedure listed in this section is a modification of the Level R, Radioactive Hazards procedure presented in the NFPA, Hazardous Materials Response Handbook [6].

*The primary objective of equipment and skin decontamination is to prevent internal contamination through ingestion or inhalation of radioactive materials and to minimize skin injury and ulceration from "beta" burns [7].*

Important Note: *Much of the decontamination process is done while the first responder is actively using an SCBA. Efforts must be made to provide change-out capability for air cylinders or fixed airline supply for personnel while they are undergoing decontamination. The person doing the decontamination and cylinder exchange must wear protective clothing, gauntlet type butyl rubber gloves, and SCBA. Care must be taken with gauntlet gloves to prevent contaminated materials from flowing down into the glove from the top. Medical gloves may be used inside of gauntlet gloves, and taping may help to prevent contamination from contacting the hands. If EPA "Level B" disposable chemical garments are available, they should be worn.[22].*

Decontamination Procedure:

The decontamination procedures presented provide basic information for decontaminating first responders at the scene of a radiological incident. Incident commanders may alter these procedures if conditions require changes.

1. A decontamination crew is assembled. It dons protective clothing (at a minimum hand and foot protection) for low level contamination, HEPA (high efficiency particulate absorption) filter masks for low level contamination and SCBAs for high levels of contamination, and lays out the decontamination areas and corridor.

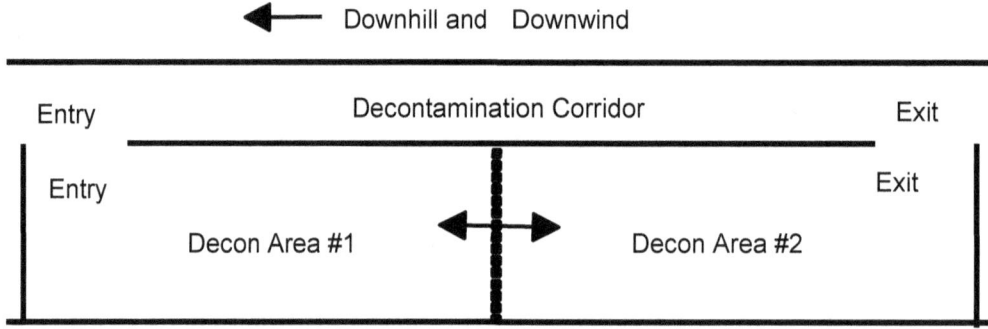

Figure 1. Decontamination Area Layout

2. The crew lays water supply lines needed for decontamination, and prepares a supply of detergent and water solution in a large clean container. Large soft scrub brushes will be positioned in the decontamination area. Scrub brushes should not be used on the skin.

3. The decontamination crew begins decontamination triage as first responders return from work.

Decontamination Triage:

Important Note: *In cases where radioactive materials are present and the level of environmental radiological exposure is manageable, it is emphasized that the contamination on the victim presents little or no danger to the responder rendering necessary first-aid even if the victim has not been fully and properly decontaminated. Proper first-aid should ALWAYS be administered [15]. It is important that life-saving procedures take precedence over decontamination.*

1. First responders suspected of being contaminated with radioactive materials will enter Decon Area #1 at a point away from the flow path of contaminated wash water.

2. Personnel are evaluated for visible signs of injury, skin, and protective equipment contamination. Note: *Medical attention takes precedence over decontamination, unless injuries are minor.* Begin decontamination procedures first on personnel that need medical attention.

3. Carefully scan personnel with a radiation monitor suitable for detecting surface contamination, TBM-3SR or equivalent. All parts of their protective clothing and equipment will be scanned, including the soles of boots. If no reading above normal background level is measured, the person can leave the decontamination area through a safe corridor.

4. Personnel found to be contaminated will begin the decontamination process.

Decontamination Process:

Warning : *No one involved in the decontamination process either personnel being decontaminated or personnel doing the decontamination work should eat, drink, or smoke while in the decontamination area. All personnel must be careful not to touch the face or other skin surfaces with contaminated hands, gloves, or other contaminated materials during the decontamination process. This is to minimize potential for ingestion and internal contamination.*

1. The contaminated first responder will enter Decon Area #1.

2. Do not remove the SCBA facepiece. The SCBA will be used throughout the decontamination process to supply safe clean air to the individual undergoing decontamination.

Note: *If the air supply must be changed during the decontamination process, and the SCBA is contaminated, the mask, associated regulator, hoses, and valves must be thoroughly flushed before changing the air supply. If it is possible that radioactive materials may be inhaled when an air supply is changed, first responders while still wearing the mask should hold their breath during the change-out procedure. Be careful not to break the mask seal. When the change-out is completed, exhale part of the breath to purge the mask and carefully inhale to insure that the system is working properly before taking a full breath. If the breathing mask must be changed, the first responder should hold their breath while changing the facepiece.*

Note: *If it is unlikely that the person being decontaminated will inhale radioactive materials during the decontamination procedure, a HEPA filter mask may be substituted for the SCBA system and mask. (A HEPA {high efficiency particulate absorption} filter cartridge or mask will remove particulate materials as small as 0.3 μm and larger with a minimum efficiency of 99.97 % [25].)*

3. For small areas of contamination on equipment or personal protective clothing, the following procedure may be used for removing radioactive particles. Apply self-adhering adhesive tape to lift removable material from surfaces. The procedure works best with dry dust type contamination. Clothing lint rollers often work well for removing contaminates. *Duct tape should not be used to remove contamination from the skin.*

4. Personnel found to be contaminated must have the contaminated components of their protective clothing and equipment scrubbed down with detergent and water. The decontamination process starts with the upper most contaminated item and progresses downward until the soles of the boot are clean. After scrubbing with the brush and detergent solution, contaminated areas are thoroughly flushed with low pressure water.

5. After preliminary decontamination is completed, first responders move to Decon Area #2 where they are carefully scanned again with a radiation detection meter. If any readings above normal background are found the person will return to Decon Area #1 and Steps 3 or 4 will be repeated as needed. The process of scanning for radioactive materials, scrubbing and flushing continues until the person's equipment is clean or it is determined that the equipment must be discarded. Note: *Throughout this procedure, the most essential concern is to minimize dose to the individual. After initial decon is completed and the equipment is still heavily contaminated, it may be more appropriate to remove the protective clothing and determine if the individual is clean.*

5. When radiological contamination has been removed, the first responder will advance out of the Decontamination Corridor and remove their protective clothing and equipment. The person's body should then be scanned for contamination.

6. In the event that complete decontamination can not be accomplished the person will advance to Decon Area #2, carefully remove as much clothing as possible, and don clean spare clothing. Efforts must be made to prevent cross contamination between the used and new clothing. The contaminated clothing that was taken off is placed in a thick wall, plastic garbage bag, sealed, and labeled for return to the station.

Doffing and Securing Radiological Contaminated PPE:

Note: *All of this doffing procedure is accomplished with the aid of a decontamination crew member. As contaminated protective clothing and equipment items are removed they are immediately placed into thick wall, plastic, garbage bags. Bags are sealed and labeled as they are filled.*

1. Remove helmet.

2. Remove the hood, if worn.

3. Doffing the SCBA tank and harness: Important Note: – *If it is possible that first responders will inhale radioactive materials, the first responders*

*should hold their breath during this operation.* A decontamination crew member will remove the air supply connection (regulator) from the SCBA mask. At a minimum, a clean HEPA filter particulate cartridge will be inserted into the mask. The first responder will exhale through the mask to purge the mask and begin breathing. Or, the SCBA mask will be removed and the first responder will immediately don, at a minimum, a HEPA filter particulate mask before inhaling. Doff the SCBA tank and harness. If the cylinder, harness, hoses, and valves were contaminated, place these items into thick wall, 6 mil (0.15 mm) or thicker, plastic garbage bags, seal, and label the bags for return to the station.

4. Remove gloves. Clean latex or thin rubber gloves may be put on at this point to keep hands clean.

5. Remove the turnout coat

6. Remove boots. If clean thin over boots are available that will easily slip through bunker pants as they are removed, they may be put on at this time to keep feet clean.

7. Remove bunker pants.

8. If over boots were put on, they should be removed and placed in a waste bag or container for contaminated materials.

9. If latex or rubber gloves were put on during step 4, they should be carefully removed and placed in a waste bag or container for contaminated materials.

10. Put on clean clothes. The person is carefully scanned again with a radioactive materials detection meter. If there are any readings of 100 cpm or higher above normal background level, the person will receive additional decontamination as follows:

The contaminated person will shower with soap and water. Hair will be shampooed. Wash in a sequence from head to toe scrubbing all body surfaces with soap and water. *Do not allow the scrubbing process to break the skin; internal radioactive materials contamination may result.* Care should be taken to insure that areas around the mouth (mustache), nostrils, and under fingernails are clean. Hair is very difficult to decontaminate because of the high oil content. Be prepared to cut hair off if necessary.

After the shower, the first responder will be checked again with the radioactive materials detection meter. If it is found that they are still contaminated, the contaminated portions should be covered to prevent dislodging and the person will be transported to a medical facility or other facility that has advanced decontamination capabilities. *Facilities having advanced CBRN decontamination capabilities should be pre-identified as a part of the emergency responder's standard operating procedures.* If personnel are found to be clean of radioactive contamination, they may proceed with normal activities.

Important Note: *Any contaminated tools carried by first responders or auxiliary equipment should also be decontaminated at the incident site. They should be scrubbed with detergent solution and flushed with water until contamination is removed before the items are taken from the Decon Area. If the items can not be decontaminated, they shall be placed in thick walled, 6 mil (0.15 mm) or thicker, plastic, garbage bags, sealed, and labeled before returning them to the station.*

Post Doffing Evaluation:

When all gear has been removed, each first responder should be checked to insure that they have not received hazardous materials contamination that was not visible when the protective clothing was being worn. If it is found that a person has been contaminated, do the following:

1. Strip any additional clothing from the body that may be contaminated.

2. Wash the contaminated body portions with copious amounts of lukewarm water and soap.

3. Cover the victim to prevent chill and further loss of body heat.

4. Provide immediate medical care, if needed.

Final Step: When all personnel have been successfully decontaminated, the decontamination crew will decontaminate each other following the steps above.

Actions Upon Returning to the Station

1. Secure apparatus at the station. If apparatus is contaminated, secure outside in an area protected from the public.

2. Secure all contaminated materials in an exterior cordoned-off area away from public access. Materials will be removed and/or salvaged by appropriate parties recommended by local, state, or federal authorities. *This process should be pre-planned based on local resources and requirements.*

Personal hygiene:

3. Shower if needed. Excess showering can be harmful. Shampoo hair. Wash in sequence from head to toe scrubbing all of the body with soap and

water. Care should be taken to insure that areas around the mouth (mustache), nostrils, under fingernails, under arms, and groin areas are clean.

4. After showering, personnel exposed to radioactive materials should be scanned again with a radioactive materials detection meter, and follow-up medical care should be provided if necessary.

# Section VI

# MULTIPLE THREAT WMD INCIDENTS

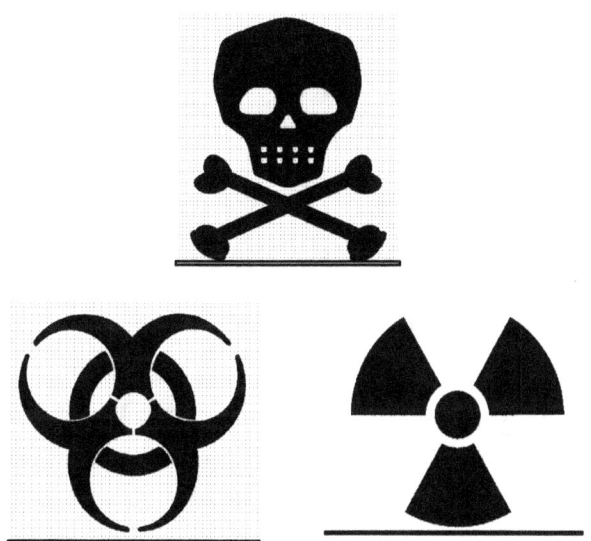

## VI. DECONTAMINATION FOR MULTIPLE WMD THREAT EXPOSURES

This section discusses decontamination processes for worst case WMD exposure scenarios. Multiple threats to life can significantly complicate first responder safety at the incident scene. Multiple threats may result from a terrorist using a combination of CBRN weapons during a single attack. However, procedures for decontamination of multiple threat attacks are not much different from the three cases discussed above. The decontamination process is simply a logical combination of the previously discussed decontamination methods.

Important Note: *An important point to remember is that decontamination for chemical agents should always be performed first, and it is typically sufficient for preliminary decontamination of biological agents. Chemical agent exposure is immediately hazardous while biological agent contamination does not generally pose an immediate threat to life, except with certain bio-toxins.*

Preliminary Decontamination for Multiple WMD Threat Exposures

The procedure listed in this section is a modification of the three procedures listed above that are based on the Level C Extreme Hazard and Level R Radioactive Hazards procedures presented in the NFPA, Hazardous Materials Response Handbook [6].

Important Note: *Much of the decontamination process is done while the first responder is actively using their SCBA. Efforts must be made to provide change-out capability for air cylinders or fixed airline supply for personnel while they are undergoing decontamination. The person doing the decontamination and cylinder exchange must wear protective clothing, gauntlet type butyl rubber gloves, and SCBA. Care must be taken with gauntlet gloves to prevent contaminated materials from flowing down into the glove from the top. Medical gloves may be used inside of gauntlet gloves, and taping may help to prevent contamination from contacting the hands.*

*If EPA "Level B" disposable chemical garments are available, they should be worn.[22].*

Important Note: *HEPA filter masks are not recommended for use during this combined decontamination procedure. Toxic gases may continue to be emitted from contaminated protective clothing and equipment during the procedure.*

Decontamination Procedure:

The decontamination procedures presented provide the basic information for decontaminating first responders at the scene of a multiple threat WMD incident. Incident Commanders may alter these procedures if conditions require changes.

1. A decontamination crew is assembled. It dons protective clothing, SCBAs, and lays out the decontamination areas and corridor.

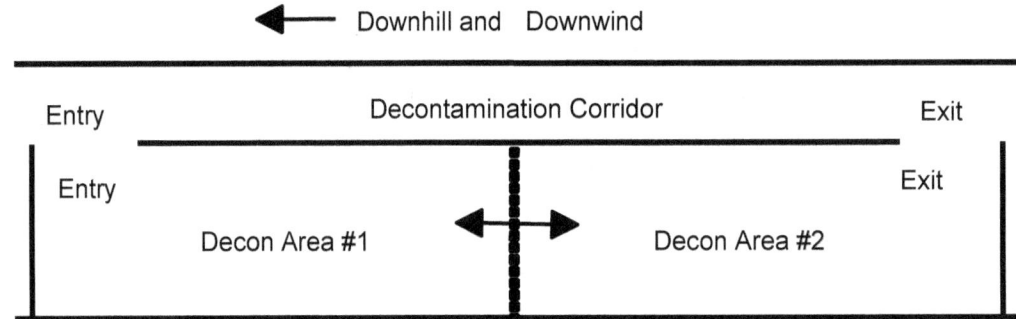

Figure 1. Decontamination area layout.

2. The crew lays water supply lines needed for decontamination, and prepares a supply of detergent and water solution in a large clean container. Large soft scrub brushes will be positioned in the decontamination area. If a soap detergent solution and brushes are not available use large volumes of low pressure water for decontamination. *Scrub brushes should not be used on the skin.*

3. The decontamination crew begins decontamination triage as first responders are returning from the incident work area.

Decontamination Triage:

Important Note: *In cases where radioactive materials are present and the level of environmental radiological exposure is manageable, it is emphasized that radiological contamination on the victim presents little or no danger to the responder rendering necessary first-aid, even if the victim has not been fully and properly decontaminated. Proper first-aid should ALWAYS be administered* [15]. *It is important that life-saving procedures take precedence over decontamination.*

1. For cases where radioactive materials may be present, carefully scan personnel with a radiation detection device suitable for detecting surface contamination. (Use a TBM-3SR meter or equivalent.) All parts of their protective clothing and equipment will be scanned, including the soles of boots. If no reading above normal background level is measured and no other contamination is observed or suspected, the person can leave the decontamination area through a safe corridor.

2. First responders suspected of being contaminated will enter Decon Area#1 at a point away from the flow path of contamination wash water.

3. Evaluate personnel for signs of chemical agent toxicity, indications of biological exposure, and scan personnel for radioactive materials contamination. Exposed skin and all personal protective clothing and equipment must be evaluated for the possibility of contamination. Decontaminate personnel exhibiting the need for medical attention first.

4. If no personnel show signs of chemical agent toxicity, but have indications that a chemical agent or radioactive material has contacted the skin or hair, decontaminate those personnel next. It should be remembered that personnel with physically damaged (cut or torn) PPE may be receiving a higher dose of chemical agent and/or radiological exposure that someone with fully intact gear.

5. If no personnel have indications of chemical agent, toxic biological agent, or radioactive material exposure to the skin or hair then, decontaminate the person having the greatest amount of contamination showing or measured on their PPE. Work down to the individual having the smallest amount of visible or measured contamination on their PPE.

6. If no personnel have health threat contamination showing or measured on their PPE, then decontaminate the first responder with the lowest air supply first. Be sure to decontaminate all personnel leaving the hot zone to insure that the chemical agents, biological agents, or radiological materials are not spread to safe areas.

Decontamination Process:

Warning :  *No one involved in the decontamination process either personnel being decontaminated or personnel doing the decontamination work should eat, drink, or smoke while in the decontamination area. All personnel must be careful not to touch the face or other skin surfaces with contaminated hands, gloves, or other contaminated materials during the decontamination process.*

1. The contaminated first responder will enter Decon Area #1.

2. Do not remove the SCBA facepiece. The SCBA will be used throughout the decontamination process to supply safe clean air to the individual undergoing decontamination.

Important Note: *If the air supply must be change during the decontamination process, the mask, associated regulator, hoses, and valves must be thoroughly flushed before changing the air supply. If it is possible that contamination or contaminated materials may be inhaled when the air supply is changed, first responders while still wearing the mask should hold their breath while the change-out is in progress. Be careful not to break the mask seal. When the change-out is completed, exhale part of the breath to purge the mask and carefully inhale to insure that the system is working properly before taking a full breath. If the breathing mask must be changed, the first responder should hold their breath while changing the facepiece.*

3. Place the helmet on the back of the neck, suspended by the neck strap. If you desire to remove the helmet, decontaminate it by flushing with water, remove it, flush the interior, and then place the helmet in an area set aside for decontaminated equipment.

4. Flush first responder downwards from head to toe with copious amounts of low pressure water. Brush with detergent solution if available. Flush the inside and outside of the helmet, hood if worn, all outside surfaces of the mask, SCBA cylinder, harness, hoses, valves, outside coat surfaces, outside surfaces (including surface folds) of coat wrist cuffs, gloves, bunker pants, and boots. *Do not use the scrub brushes to clean human skin.*

5. Tools carried by first responders must also be flushed with water and washed to remove contamination.

6. When all visible contamination has been removed, the first responder will advance to Decon Area #2 where they are carefully scanned again with a radioactive materials detection meter. If any radiation reading is above the normal background level, the person returns to Decon Area #1 and will receive further decontamination.

7. Contaminated components of the protective clothing and equipment ensemble will be scrubbed down again and flushed with low pressure water. The decontamination process starts with the upper most contaminated item and progresses downward until the soles of the boot are clean.

8. The process of scanning for radioactive materials, scrubbing and flushing continues until the person's equipment is clean or it is determined that the equipment must be discarded.

9. The first responder then advances again to Decon Area #2 to remove their protective clothing and equipment.

Doff and Securing Decontaminated PPE:

1. Remove helmet.

2. Remove gloves.

3. Remove the air supply connection (regulator) from the SCBA mask, and doff the SCBA tank and harness. If the cylinder, harness, hoses, and valves were contaminated, place these items in thick walled, 6 mil (0.15 mm) or thicker, garbage bags and seal the bags for return to the station. Label the bags to indicate the contents.

4. Remove the hood, if worn.

5. Remove the SCBA mask

6. Remove the turnout coat

7. Remove boots.

8. Remove bunker pants.

9. If circumstances permit, bag all additional protective clothing and equipment that were contaminated. Place items in thick walled, 6 mil (0.15 mm) or thicker, garbage bags and seal the bags for return to the station. Label the bags with the person's name and the contents of the bag.

Emergency Field Decontamination of Equipment

In the event that an apparatus crew must be immediately dispatched to another incident, additional measures must be taken to insure that their personal protective clothing and equipment have been decontaminated. First, insure that the PPE is not contaminated by radioactive materials. This is done by carefully scanning the equipment with a radioactive materials detection meter. When the gear has been determined to be clean of radiological materials, it should be washed down with one of the detoxification solutions listed in Section I - 3.2, page 10 and discussed in the Section III, page 31, entitled, Decontamination by Chemical Methods – Oxidation and Hydrolysis. The chlorite based chemical solutions and high pH solutions are suitable for the decontamination process. Rugged plastic pump sprayers used for gardening have been found to be suitable for dispensing decontamination solutions. After the decontamination chemicals have been applied and allowed to stay in place for the specified time, the equipment should be thoroughly flushed with water.

Note: *It is important to remember that some decontamination solutions may cause a level of deterioration in the protective equipment.*

Doffing and Securing Radiological Contaminated PPE:

Note: *All of this doffing procedure is accomplished with the aid of a decontamination crew member. As contaminated protective clothing and equipment items are removed they are immediately placed into thick wall, plastic, garbage bags. Bags are sealed and labeled as they are filled.*

1. Remove helmet.

2. Remove the hood, if worn.

3. Doffing the SCBA tank and harness: Important Note: - *If it is possible that first responders will inhale radioactive materials, the first responders should hold their breath during this operation.* A decontamination crew member will remove the air supply connection (regulator) from the SCBA mask. At a minimum, a clean HEPA filter particulate cartridge will be inserted into the mask. The first responder will exhale through the mask to purge the mask and begin breathing. Or, the SCBA mask will be removed and the first responder will immediately don, at a minimum, a HEPA filter

particulate mask before inhaling.  Doff the SCBA tank and harness.  If the cylinder, harness, hoses, and valves were contaminated, place these items into thick walled, 6 mil (0.15 mm) or thicker, plastic garbage bags, seal, and label the bags for return to the station.

4. Remove gloves.

5. Remove the turnout coat.

6. Remove boots.

8. Remove bunker pants.

9. The person is carefully scanned again with a radioactive materials detection meter.  If clean, they will put on clean clothes.  If there are any readings above normal background, the person will be receive additional decontamination as follows:

The contaminated person will shower with soap and water.  Hair will be shampooed.  Wash in a sequence from head to toe scrubbing all body surfaces with soap and water using a soft brush.  *Do not allow the scrubbing process to break the skin; internal radioactive materials contamination may result.*  Care should be taken to insure that areas around the mouth (mustache), nostrils, and under fingernails are clean.

After the shower, the first responder will be checked again with the radioactive materials detection meter.  If it is found that they are still contaminated, the contaminated portions should be covered to prevent dislodging and the person will be transported to a medical facility or other facility that has advanced decontamination capabilities.  *Facilities having advanced CBRN decontamination capabilities should be pre-identified as a part of the emergency responder's standard operating procedures.*  If personnel are found to be clean of radioactive contamination, they may proceed with normal activities.

Important Note: *Any contaminated tools carried by first responders or auxiliary equipment should also be decontaminated at the incident site.  They should be scrubbed with detergent solution and flushed with water until contamination is removed before the items are taken from the Decon Area.  If the items can not be decontaminated, they shall be placed in thick walled, 6 mil (0.15 mm) or thicker, plastic, garbage bags, sealed, and labeled before returning them to the station.*

Post Doffing Evaluation:

When all gear has been removed, each first responder must be checked to insure that the toxic agents did not contact the skin or hair.  If it is found that the person has additional contamination, do the following:

1. Blot any chemical agent from the skin.

2. Strip any additional clothing from the body that may be contaminated.

3. Flush the body with copious amounts of water. Soap and water is better.

4. Cover the victim to prevent chill and further loss of body heat.

5. Provide immediate medical care.

Final Step: When all personnel have been successfully decontaminated, the decontamination crew will decontaminate each other following the steps above.

Actions Upon Returning to the Station

1. Secure apparatus on the exterior of station.

2. Secure all contaminated materials in an exterior cordoned-off area away from public access.

Personal hygiene:

3. Strip completely and place all clothing, protective and personal, in plastic bags. Seal and label the bags. Place bags in exterior cordoned-off area.

4. Shower. Shampoo hair. Wash in sequence from head to toe scrubbing all of the body with soap and water. Care should be taken to insure that areas around the mouth (mustache), nostrils, under fingernails, under arms, and groin areas are clean.

Note: *Research of fire fighters using turnout gear in simulated chemical weapons agent environments showed that moist areas of the body (e.g. groin and under arms) are most susceptible to some chemical agents [23].*

5. Personnel exposed to chemical agents should receive a medical examination.

# Section VII

# POST-INCIDENT EQUIPMENT DECONTAMINATION

## VII. POST-INCIDENT EQUIPMENT DECONTAMINATION

Equipment and materials that were field decontaminated may still contain life threatening concentrations of agents or radioactive materials after being returned to the station. These materials must be further evaluated, receive further decontamination and cleaning, or disposed of if they are not usable or recoverable. *In the event that the equipment can not be immediately decontaminated or disposed of by a professional environmental control team and the equipment must be put back into service, additional decontamination and cleaning is required.* This section of the document discusses issues associated with follow up decontamination of equipment, and it provides options that may be used for this more advance decontamination process. Many of these methods are relatively simple to accomplish; however, it must be remembered that the decontamination processes must be carried out with extreme caution. *Maximum protection must be provided for all personnel involved in final detoxification and decontamination of the equipment.* In addition, any decontamination work conducted in by fire departments or other first responders must also consider the environmental impact of the decontamination process on the community where the work is being carried out. The following are some of the issues to be considered:

- Personnel and community safety is number one.
- The decontamination process must be carried out in a highly controlled manner.
- If evaporative or thermal methods are used to decontaminate equipment, it must be done in an area where there is no harmful exposure to people or the environment down wind of the activity.
- If chemical methods are used, contaminated liquids and other decontamination byproducts must be contained and collected to prevent the possibility of spreading contamination.

For chemical agent and biological decontamination the following procedures may be used:

*Before conducting these processes, be sure to address local, state, and federal regulations for conducting these types of decontamination operations. These regulations should be identified and prepared for as a part of pre-planning for CBRN operations.*

Important Note: *All procedures outlined in this section shall be accomplished by personnel wearing at a minimum EPA "Level B" protective garments and SCBAs [22]. Disposable garment systems are preferred.*

Chemical and biological warfare agents can be rendered harmless through physical methods using heat and ultraviolet radiation. Many chemical agents are non-persistent or are semi-persistent. These agents can usually be easily removed simply by evaporation followed by washing using normal laundry procedures. Many biological agents can be destroyed by the application of dry heat or stream heat. Even allowing equipment to dry while exposed to solar ultraviolet radiation has a disinfectant effect on some biological agents; however this method is not recommended since it is highly variable [1]. The most productive physical methods for chemical and biological agent decontamination are listed below.

## PHYSICAL METHODS FOR CHEMICAL WARFARE AGENT DECONTAMINATION

Expose the chemical agent contaminated materials to the following conditions until dry:

Hang contaminated materials (equipment, tools, and protective clothing, etc.) in a vented compartment that can be heated to 40 °C (105 °F). Be sure that gases vented from the compartment do not endanger personnel, the public, or the environment near the decontamination process. If the gases are vented high above the ground, atmospheric dilution will typically reduce toxicity of the vented gases as they travel away from the evaporation compartment. Important Note: *Care must be taken to insure that no one is directly down wind and near the evaporation compartment.*

After the materials have been dried and the evaporation process is completed, the heat is turned off and the materials are bagged up in thick wall, 6 mil (0.15 mm) or thicker, plastic, garbage bags, seal in the bags and transported to be washed. Normal laundry wash cycles may be used that are specified for protective clothing laundry processes; however, wash solutions having an alkaline pH of 8 or 9 will do a better job of finishing the decontamination process. The alkaline wash will take advantage of chemical detoxification of any remaining residue.

## PHYSICAL METHODS FOR BIOLOGICAL WARFARE AGENT DECONTAMINATION

### DRY HEAT METHOD:

- Expose biologically contaminated materials to one of the following temperature/time conditions [1][26]:

> *180 °C (356 °F) for ................30 minutes*
> *170 °C (340 °F) for .............1 hour*
> *160 °C (320 °F) for.............. 2 hours.*
> *150 °C (300 °F) for .............2.5 hours*

Some fire training facilities have live fire training compartments that may be adapted for the above dry heat method of decontamination. It is critical that all components and parts of the materials being decontaminated reach the recommended dry heat temperature, and they must be maintained at the given temperature for at least the specified time period.

### STEAM HEAT METHOD, AUTOCLAVING:

- Expose contaminated materials to a pressure of 1 atmosphere (15 psi or 103 kPa) above normal atmospheric pressure with a steam temperature of 121 °C (250 °F) and a decontamination exposure time of 20 minutes [26].

No field expedient method has been identified to replicate the steam heat method. However, many medical and some research facilities have large autoclaves that could be used for biological agent decontamination.

## CHEMICAL METHODS FOR CHEMICAL AND BIOLOGICAL WARFARE AGENT DECONTAMINATION

The most often recommended method for decontamination of materials exposed to biological agents using chemical methods is associated with the use of chlorine containing solutions. Manufacturers of fibers and fabric materials used in the manufacturer of fire service protective clothing materials do not recommend that their materials be exposed to laundry detergents, bleaches, or disinfectants containing chlorine. Particularly, fabrics containing Kevlar® fibers are susceptible to loss of strength after exposure to chlorine. However, laboratory tests have shown that a single short time period exposure to a common commercial household chlorine bleach (6% sodium hypochlorite solution) will not seriously degrade fabrics containing Kevlar®, and it will decontaminate garments exposed to all known biological agents. Therefore, the following procedures may be used in emergency situations to decontaminate fire service PPE using a commercial household chlorine bleach solution [24][26]:

## EMERGENCY DECONTAMINATION USING 6 % CHLORINE BLEACH

Warning: *This treatment is for emergency decontamination only and should be used only one time on materials containing Kevlar®.*

- Completely soak the protective clothing and equipment for one minute in undiluted Ultra Clorox® regular bleach or equivalent that contains a 6 % sodium hypochlorite solution.
- Do not dilute the manufacturer's bleach solution with water, as is normally done.
- After the one minute soak in ultra chlorine bleach, immediately rinse the protective clothing with large quantities of tepid water.

Note: *Some materials may show a change in color.*

Warning: *For fabrics made with Kevlar®, repeated exposures to chlorine containing solutions will result in serious loss of material strength and will cause the protective clothing systems to fail when in normal use.*

Effectiveness: The above decontamination procedure will inactivate 99.8 % of *anthrax* spores in one minute and will completely inactivate *E. coli* over the same time period [25].

# DECONTAMINATION USING 6 % CHLORINE BLEACH

Use on fire fighters' protective clothing and equipment that does not contain materials that are seriously degraded by exposure to chlorine solutions.

This process may be used on protective equipment that does not contain Kevlar® and has firm or hard equipment surfaces. Examples: helmets, rubber boots, some gloves, SCBA tanks and harness frames, masks, rubber hoses, and external regulator surfaces.

Warning: *Check with your SCBA manufacturer for decontamination procedures for internal components of SCBA regulators and masks.*

- Completely soak the protective clothing and equipment for 15 minutes in a household bleach (sodium hypochlorite) solution that has been diluted to produce a 0.26 % (1:22) bleach solution.
- After the 15 minute soak in the 1:22 bleach solution, immediately rinse the protective clothing and equipment with large quantities of tepid water.

Effectiveness: The above decontamination procedure will inactivate 100 % of *anthrax* spores exposed to the treatment [25].

# Section VIII

# SUMMARY

# SUMMARY

This document has been prepared to provide the first responder with a basic aid for conducting decontamination processes in the event they are needed. As mentioned earlier, this document has attempted to address the primary basic elements of decontamination, but does not address all possible conditions and situations. It is the responsibility of the first responders at the scene to execute decontamination procedures appropriate for the incident. It is recommended that all first responders be trained in decontamination processes and that they conduct exercises to help validate their procedures. In addition, first responders should attempt to stay current with new information concerning CBRN operations and decontamination.

A brief discussion of cold weather decontamination was provided in Section I. More detailed information can be found in a recently published document by SBCCOM, "Guidelines for Cold Weather Mass Decontamination During a Terrorist Chemical Agent Incident." Additional information published by SBCCOM on mass decontamination may be useful, "Guidelines for Mass Casualty Decontamination During a Terrorist Chemical Agent Incident."

The success of the decontamination effort is greatly influenced by how well first responders protect themselves and how quickly they can effectively conduct decontamination procedures. With large numbers of casualties the challenge to first responders is greatly increased. However, training and realistic exercises can significantly improve the probability of success. First responders should share their procedures, training, and exercises with neighboring fire and rescue organizations.

Decontamination of first responder's personal protective equipment (PPE) is a major component of this document. Short term and extended operations are dependent on the use of this equipment (PPE) and the availability to replace it when needed. Some fire and rescue organizations can provide their personnel with two sets of equipment; however, most fire and rescue organizations do not have these resources. Therefore, it is important that first responders know how to safely and effectively decontaminate their PPE after exposure to a suspected or known CBRN environment. Following this aid for decontamination will serve to not only clean the PPE, but also will make the equipment available for other emergency incidents.

# REFERENCES

[1] Office of the Surgeon General, Medical Aspects of Chemical and Biological Warfare, Textbook of Military Medicine, Hurst, Charles G., M.D., Chapter 15 Decontamination, Department of the Army, 1997

[2] National Fire Protection Association, NFPA 1971 Standard on Protective Ensemble for Structural Fire Fighting," 2000 Edition, Quincy, MA.

[3] National Fire Protection Association, NFPA 1851 Standard on Selection, Care, and Maintenance of Structural Fire Fighting Protective Ensembles," 2001 Edition, Quincy, MA.

[4] TRI/Environmental, Inc., Decontamination of Structural Fire Fighting Protective Clothing and Equipment, Final Report, Contract No. EMW-92-C-3987, United States Fire Administration, Emmitsburg, MD, December 1994.

[5] Emergency Response to Terrorism, Job Aid, The Federal Emergency Management Agency, United States Fire Administration, National Fire Academy, and United States Department of Justice Office of Justice Programs, Edition 1.0, May 2000.

[6] Smeby, Charles L., Jr., Editor, Hazardous Materials Response Handbook, Third Edition National Fire Protection Association, Quincy, MA, 1997.

[7] Department of the Navy, BUMEDINST 6470.10A, Initial Management Of Irradiated Or Radioactively Contaminated Personnel, United States Navy, Bureau of Medicine and Surgery, Washington, DC, 1998.

[8] Hawley, Gessner, G., The Condensed Chemical Dictionary, Eight Edition, Van Nostrand Reinhold Company, New York, 1971.

[9] Trapp, R., The Detoxification and Natural Degradation of Chemical Warfare Agents, Stockholm, Sweden; Stockholm International Peace Research Institute (SIPRI); pp. 44 – 75, 1985.

[10] Yurow, H.W., Decontamination methods for HD, GB, and VX: A literature survey, Aberdeen Proving Ground, MD: Army Armament Research and Development Command; Chemical Systems Laboratory, AD-B057349L, 1981.

[11] Booz-Allen & Hamilton Inc. and Science Applications International Corporation, Hazmat Technician Decontamination Procedures, Module 10, Domestic Preparedness Training Program, V7.0 CD-ROM, 1998.

[12] Centers for Disease Control and Prevention, Special Pathogens Branch, Teaching and Prevention Materials, "Infection Control for Viral Haemorrhagic Fevers in the African Health Care Setting," WWW.cdc.gov/ncidod/dvrd/spb/mnpages/vhfmanual.htm, 2002

[13] American Association of Textile Chemists and Colorists, AATCC Standard Test Method 135, Dimensional Changes in Automatic Home Laundering of Woven and Knit Fabrics, Technical Manual, Research Triangle Park, NC, 2000

[14] American Society for Testing and Materials, ASTM D5034 Standard Test Method for Breaking Strength and Elongation of Textile Fabrics(Grab Test), Annual Book of ASTM Standards, Vol. 07.02, West Conshohocken, PA, 2000.

[15] Armed Forces Radiobiology Research Institute (AFRRI), Medical Effects of Ionizing Radiation, Military/Medical Operations Office, (MEIR) CD-ROM Course, Bethesda, MD, 1999.

[15] 2000 Emergency Response Guidebook, A Guidebook for First Responders During the Initial Phase of a Dangerous Goods/Hazardous Materials Incident, U.S. Department of Transportation (DOT), Washington, DC.

[17] United States Marine Corps, Nuclear, Biological & Chemical Warfare Defense, Basic Officer Course, Marine Corps Combat Development Command, Quantico, VA, 1999.

[18] Occupational Safety and Health Administration, OSHA Technical Manual, Section VIII, Chapter 1, Chemical Protective Clothing, www.osha-slc.gov/dts/osta/otm/otm_viii/otm_viii_1.html, 2002

[19] McIntosh, Roger G.; Dousa, Todd A.; Weyandt, Timothy B.; Toxic Chemical Training Course for Medical Support Personnel, Instructors Guide, Decontamination and the Management of Contaminated Casualties, Science Application International Corporation, 1998.

[20] van Hooidonk C., CW agents and the skin: Penetration and decontamination. In: Proceedings of the International Symposium on Protection Against Chemical Warfare Agents; June 6-9, 1983; Stockholm, Sweden, National Defense Research Institute.

[21] Papirmeister, B., Feister, A., Robinson, S., and Ford, R., Medical Defense Against Mustard Gas: Toxic Mechanisms and Pharmacological Implications, Boca Raton, FL: CRC Press; 1991: 92.

[22] Environmental Protection Agency, Standard Operating Safety Guides, Office of Emergency and Remedial Response, Environmental Response Team, U.S. Government Printing Office, 748-159/20417, 1990.

[23]  U.S. Army SBCCOM Domestic Preparedness Chemical Team, Guidelines for Incident Commander's Use of Firefighter Protective Ensemble (FFPE) with Self-Contained Breathing Apparatus (SCBS) for Rescue Operations During a Terrorist Chemical Agent Incident, Edgewood, MD, 1999.

[24]  Centers for Disease Control and Prevention, CDC:  SPB: Teaching Materials:  VHF Precautions Manual, U.S. Department of Health and Human Services, http://www.cdc.gov/ncidod/dvrd/spb/mnpages/vhfmanual.htm, 2002

[25]  Hawley, Robert J. and Eitzen, Edward M. Jr., Biological Weapons – A Primer for Microbiologests, Annual Review of Microbiology, 55:235-253, 2001.

[26]  Perkins, John J., M.S., LL.D., F.R.S.H., Principles and Methods of Sterilization in Health Sciences, Second Edition, Eighth Printing, Charles C. Thomas Publishing, Springfield, IL., 1983.

[27]  National Council on Radiation Protection and Measurements, Management of Terrorist Events Involving Radioactive Material, NCRP Report No. 138, Bethesda, MD, October 2001.

[28]  Ionizing Radiation Series No. 1, Radiation Protection Program Publication, U.S. Environmental Protection Agency EPA 402-F98-009, May 1998, http://www.epa.gov/radiation/ionize.htm

[29]  Canberra Dover (formally Aptec-NRC), UDR-13, PED-13A Radiac Set Data Sheets, Dover, NJ, 2002

[30]  $T_A$ Technical Associates, Model TBM-3SR Surface Contamination Monitor Manuel, Technical Associates, Canoga Park, www.tech-associates.com, CA 2002

[31]  A Fact Sheet on the Health Effects from Ionizing Radiation, Ionizing Radiation Series No. 2, Radiation Protection Program Publication, U.S. Environmental Protection Agency EPA 402-F98-010, May 1998, http://www.epa.gov/radiation/ionize.htm

[32]  Department of Defense, Office of Civil Defense, Personal and Family Survival, Civil Defense Adult Education Course Manual, SM 3-11-A, Washington, DC, 1966.

[33]  Transportation Emergency Preparedness Program (TEPP), Radiological Incident Response, Part 2, Basic Radiological Orientation Personal, Module 2; and Personal Safety, Module 4; Student Workbook.

# APPENDIX – A

Other methods used for CWA and BWA decontamination.

Information supplied by Dupont Advanced Fiber Systems:

The following disinfecting products were tested to determine if they would degrade the properties of aramid thermal protective clothing materials. A memo provided by the Dupont Advanced Fiber Systems department that contained a list of acceptable biological disinfecting products had the following introductory statement:

"The following products were tested or reviewed and were determined not to impact the thermal properties or fibers of Nomex ® when used at recommended dilutions. The effectiveness of the disinfecting solution was not examined. Other similar products may also be acceptable." Important Note: *It was recommended that protective clothing materials that are treated with the listed disinfecting products should be washed immediately following the disinfectant treatment.*

## "CAVACIDE"

Mfg. Micaro Asceptic Products, Chicago, IL
Tested
Active ingredients: Quaternary ammonium chloride, isopropyl alcohol, and detergent.

## "IDO DISINFECTANT"

Mfg. Winsol Laboratories, Seattle, WA
Chemically reviewed
Active ingredients: Iodophor complex and phosphoric acid

## "MULTIWASH"

Mfg. EMS Products Corp., Las Vegas, NV
Chemically reviewed
Active ingredients: Nonoxynol 9 and iodophor complex

## "PURSUE GERMICIDAL CONCENTRATE"

Mfg. Amway Commercial Products, Ada, MI
Chemically reviewed
Active ingredients: Dimethyl benzyl ammonium chlorides and ethyl alcohol

"QT" & "QT1000"

Mfg. S. I. Inc., Morristown, NJ
Chemically reviewed
Active ingredients: Alkyl dimethyl benzalkonium chloride, alkyl ethyl benzalkonium chloride, and bis-tributylin oxide


"SPRITZ"

Mfg. Alda Pharmaceuticals Inc.
Chemically reviewed
Active ingredients: Ethanol, o-phenylphenol, chorhexidine gluconate, benzalkonium chloride, nonoxynol-9


"UNICIDE 128" & UNICIDE 256"

Mfg. Brulin Corp., Indianapolis, IN
Chemically reviewed
Active Ingredients: Ammonium chlorides


# MODEC DECON FORMULATION

Another decontamination product that may be used for decontaminating both chemical and biological agents has been developed by Sandia National Laboratories. Important Note: *This aqueous foam decontamination product has not been evaluated for its potential for damaging fire fighters' protective clothing and equipment.* Industry has planned research to evaluate the impact of the foam on thermal protective clothing and equipment, and it is expected that the work will be completed by January 2003. However, this product will likely be an important decontamination agent in the event of future chemical and/or biological terrorist attacks. The following are excerpts from the abstract of the technical report for the foam:

Report reference:

Modec, Inc., Formulations for the Decontamination and Mitigation of CB Warfare Agents, Toxic Hazardous Materials, Viruses, Bacteria and Bacterial Spores, MOD2001-1008-M, Denver, CO, February 2001.

"A non-toxic, non-corrosive aqueous foam with enhanced physical stability for the rapid mitigation and decontamination of chemical and biological warfare (CBW) agents and toxic hazardous materials has been developed at Sandia National Laboratories." "Experimental results have show effective decontamination of both chemical warfare (CW) and biological warfare (BW) agent simulatnts and live agents on contaminated surfaces and in solution.

Testing had also shown that the foam decontaminates thickened agent simulants as well." "Additional tests indicate that the formulation may be effective as a universal decontaminant on a variety of toxic industrial materials and other hazardous bacteria, viruses and materials such as hydrocarbon based compounds as well." "Modec, Inc. of Denver Colorado was selected by the Department of Energy to commercialize the invention pursuant to License No. 00-C00872."

## APPENDIX - B

### Ionizing Radiation Measurement Units and Conversions

The contents of this appendix are based on information found in reference [27].

The numerical units used in literature to describe radiation exposures and the measurement units used by radiation detection meters can be confusing. This appendix has been prepared to assist the first responder with understanding the terminology and units associated with radiological measurements.

There are two terms that are primarily used to describe ionizing radiation exposures, these are:

1) absorbed dose
2) effective dose.

The absorbed dose is a measure of ionizing radiation absorbed by a material. (energy absorbed per unit mass)

The effective dose is a measure of biologic effectivity of an exposure to a given quantity of ionizing radiation. This quantity is a unit of measure that is mathematically derived from the measured absorbed dose. Several other terms have also been used to describe effective dose, they are: *ambient dose equivalent, equivalent dose, and dose equivalent.*

Both of the above terms are used to describe the potential for ionizing radiation health threats to humans, although they have somewhat different meanings.

### COMMONLY USED MEASUREMENT UNITS

|  | Conventional Units | New SI Units |
|---|---|---|
| Absorbed Dose: | rad<br>(radiation absorbed dose) | Gy<br>(gray) |
| Effective Dose: | rem<br>(roentgen equivalent man) | Sv<br>(sievert) |

In the above units, use the following conversions to translate units:

The basic rule recommended for conversion between conventional radiation units is:

For Gamma and X-rays:

1 rad = 1 rem and 1 rem = 1 roentgen (R) and all are considered to be equivalent.

Meters for measuring ionizing radiation may be found using any of the above units of measurement. In addition, meters that measure low levels of ionizing radiation may include the units micro (μ) and milli (m) in combination with radiation measurement, e.g., rem or Sv. The term roentgen is often abbreviated using the capital letter R.

Examples of this usage are:

Normal background radiation is about 10 μR/h to 20 μR/h (micro-roentgens per hour) which is equivalent to 0.01 mR/h to 0.02 mR/h (milli-roentgens per hour).

$$10 \ \mu R/h \ = \ 0.01 \ mR/h$$

$$1 \ (\mu) \ micro \ unit \ = \ 0.000001 \ units \ or \ 1/1,000,000 \ units$$
$$1 \ (m) \ milli \ unit \ = \ 0.001 \ units \ or \ 1/1,000 \ units$$

Conversions between conventional units and SI units are:

$$Absorbed \ Dose \ - \ 100 \ rad \ = \ 1 \ Gy \ (gray)$$

$$Effective \ Dose \ - \ 100 \ rem \ = \ 1 \ Sv \ (sievert)$$

The following table provides unit conversions for conventional units to SI units:

Conversions for absorbed dose:

| 0.001 rad | = 1 mrad | = 0.01 mGy | |
|-----------|----------|------------|--------|
| 0.01 rad | = 10 mrad | = 0.1 mGy | |
| 0.1 rad | = 100 mrad | = 1 mGy | = 0.001 Gy |
| 1 rad | = 1,000 mrad | = 10 mGy | = 0.01 Gy |
| 10 rad | | = 100 mGy | = 0.1 Gy |
| 100 rad | | = 1,000 mGy | = 1 Gy |
| 1,000 rad | | | = 10 Gy |

Conversions for effective dose:

| 0.001 rem | = 1 mrem | = 0.01 mSv | |
|-----------|----------|------------|--------|
| 0.01 rem | = 10 mrem | = 0.1 mSv | |
| 0.1 rem | = 100 mrem | = 1 mSv | = 0.001 Sv |
| 1 rem | = 1,000 mrem | = 10 mSv | = 0.01 Sv |
| 10 rem | | = 100 mSv | = 0.1 Sv |
| 100 rem | | = 1,000 mSv | = 1 Sv |
| 1,000 rem | | | = 10 Sv |

# GLOSSARY

Acute Dose:

Energy absorbed as a result of a relatively large amount of ionizing radiation (100 rad or more) over a short period of time.

Acute Exposure:

An exposure, often intense, over a relatively short period of time.

Acute Radiation Syndrome (ARS):

A broad term used to describe a range of signs and symptoms that reflect severe damage to specific organ systems that can lead to death within hours or several weeks.

Background Radiation:

The radiation in our natural environment, including cosmic rays and radiation from the naturally radioactive elements, both inside and outside the bodies of living creatures. It is also called natural radiation. Human-made sources of radioactivity contribute to total background radiation levels. (5 to 30 $\mu$R/h or 350 to 500 mrem/y)

Chemical Agent:

There are five classes of chemical agents, all of which produce incapacitation, serious injury, or death. (1) nerve agents, (2) blister agents, (3) blood agents, (4) choking agents, (5) irritating agents. A chemical substance used in military operations is intended to kill, seriously injure, or incapacitate people through its physiological effects.

Cold Zone:

The "Support Zone," the outermost part of the incident site, considered a non-contaminated or clean area. Support equipment and the command post are located in the "Cold Zone" zone, traffic is restricted to authorized response personnel. Normal work clothes are appropriate within this zone, potentially contaminated personnel clothing, equipment, and samples are not permitted, but are left in the "Warm Zone" until they are decontaminated or made safe for transport.

Contamination:

> When a chemical, biological, or radiological material is not located where it should be, particularly if its presence can be harmful. Although often contamination is on surfaces, it can also be airborne.

Counts Per Minute (CPM):

> The number of events observed by a radiation detector in one minute. Used to measure activity when converted to disintegrations per minute (dpm). Contamination is measured in CPM or DPM per unit area.

External Exposure:

> An exposure received from a chemical or biological agent or a source of ionizing radiation outside of the human body.

Gross Decontamination:

> Initial decontamination to remove large amounts of contaminates.

Hot Zone:

> The "Exclusion Zone," the innermost of three work zone areas at an incident, is the physical area where contamination could occur. All people entering the "Hot Zone" must wear prescribed levels of protection, and they must follow procedures established to enter, work in the area, and exit the zone.

Internal Exposure:

> An exposure received from a chemical or biological agent or a source of ionizing radiation from inside of the human body. The source has been inhaled, ingested, or absorbed into the body.

Ionizing radiation (ionization):

> Energy in the form of particles or rays emitted from a radioactive (unstable) atom. Ionizing radiation has enough energy to cause ionization in atoms. Ionization is the process of adding one or more electrons to, or removing one or more electrons from, atoms or molecules, thereby creating ions. High temperatures, electrical discharges, chemical reactions, and nuclear radiation are possible causes of ionization.

Mass Decontamination:

> Decontamination process used on large numbers of contaminated victims.

Nuclear Incident:

An event in which a nuclear material is used as a terrorist weapon. There are three fundamentally different threats in the area of nuclear terrorism: (1) the use, or threatened use, of a nuclear bomb, (2) the detonation of a conventional explosive incorporating nuclear materials, a dirty bomb RDD (Radiological Dispersal Device), and (3) a simple radiological device, SRD.

Site Safety Plan:

Established policies and procedures for protecting the health and safety of response personnel during all operations conducted at an incident. It contains information about the known or suspected hazards, routine and special safety procedures that must be followed and other instructions for safeguarding the health of the responders. The plan is written and posted at the site.

Size-up:

The rapid mental evaluation of the factors that influence an incident. Size-up is the first step in determining a course of action.

Terrorism:

As defined by the FBI, "the unlawful use of force against persons or property to intimidate or coerce a government, the civilian population, or any segment thereof, in the furtherance of political or social objectives," This definition includes three elements: (1) Terrorist activities are illegal and involve the use of force. (2) The actions are intended to intimidate or coerce. (3) The actions are committed in support of political or social objectives.

Toxins:

Toxic substances of natural origin produced by an animal, plant, or microbe. They differ from chemical substances in that they are not manmade. Toxins may include botulism, ricin, and mycotoxins.

Vesicants:

Chemical agents, also called blister agents, which cause severe burns to eyes, skin, and tissues of the respiratory tract. Mustard and lewisite are examples of vesicant agents.

Warm Zone:

Located between the "Hot Zone" and the "Cold Zone" and is also known as the "Contamination Reduction Zone." This is the area that provides a transition between contaminated areas and the uncontaminated areas. The "Warm Zone" provides a buffer to further reduce the probability of the cold zone becoming contaminated or being affected by other existing hazards. Decontamination takes place in a portion of the "Warm Zone."

Weapon of Mass Destruction (WMD):

(1) Any explosive, incendiary, poison gas, bomb, grenade, or rocket having a propellant charge of more than four ounces, missile having an explosive or incendiary charge of more than one quarter ounce, or mine or device similar to the above
(2) Poison gas.
(3) Any weapon involving a disease organism.
(4) Any weapon designed to release radiation at a level dangerous to human life.

# INDEX

Notes:

Notes: